UI

PRENTICE-HALL

FOUNDATIONS OF IMMUNOLOGY SERIES

Abraham Osler and Leon Weiss, Editors

THE IMMUNOBIOLOGY OF TRANSPLANTATION
Rupert Billingham and Willys Silvers

THE CELLS AND TISSUES OF THE IMMUNE SYSTEM
Leon Weiss

PROGRESS IN TRANSPLANTATION

1970

REAWAKENED INTEREST IN HETEROGRAFTS THROUGH ALS

HUMAN HEART GRAFTS

HUMAN LIVER GRAFTS

1965 HL-A LOCUS IN MAN

ORGAN GRAFTING IN SMALL MAMMALS

MIXED LYMPHOCYTE INTERACTION

IMMUNOSUPPRESSIVE EFFECT OF ALS; TISSUE MATCHING AND TYPING

SUCCESSFUL RENAL HOMOGRAFTS IN MAN WITH IMMUNOSUPPRESSIVE DRUGS

SUCCESSFUL RENAL HOMOGRAFTS IN DOGS WITH 6-MP

IN VITRO ACTIVITY OF SENSITIZED LYMPHOCYTES

1960 IMMUNOSUPPRESSIVE EFFECT OF 6-MP IN RABBITS

TRANSPLANTATION IMMUNITY A FORM OF DELAYED HYPERSENSITIVITY

DIRECT REACTION; TRANSFER REACTION

GRAFT VS. HOST REACTIONS — CONCEPT OF PERIPHERAL SENSITIZATION

PRESENCE OF IMMUNOLOGICALLY COMPETENT CELLS IN BLOOD

ELICITATION OF TRANSPLANTATION IMMUNITY WITH CELL EXTRACTS

1955 TRANSFER OF SENSITIVITY TO HOMOGRAFTS WITH REGIONAL NODE CELLS

TUMOR SPECIFIC ANTIGENS

IMMUNOLOGIC TOLERANCE; RADIATION CHIMERAS

IMMUNOLOGIC NATURE OF ENHANCEMENT

STUDIES ON RENAL HOMOGRAFTS IN DOGS

PROLONGATION OF HOMOGRAFT SURVIVAL IN RABBITS BY { CORTISONE / WHOLE BODY IRRADIATION }

1950 GENETICS OF H-2 LOCUS OF MOUSE

ANALYSIS OF RED CELL CHIMERISM IN CATTLE

CRYOPROTECTIVE EFFECT OF GLYCEROL

IMMUNOLOGIC NATURE OF SKIN HOMOGRAFT REJECTION

1940 IMMUNOGENETIC BASIS OF TUMOR TRANSPLANTATION — BLOOD BANKS

TRANSFUSIONS COMMONPLACE

SEROLOGY OF HOMOGRAFT REACTION

INITIATION OF ANALYSIS OF ENHANCEMENT OR "XYZ" EFFECT

1930

1920

GENETIC BASIS OF TUMOR TRANSPLANTATION — DIRECT BLOOD TRANSFUSIONS

SUSPECTED ROLE OF LYMPHOCYTES IN GRAFT REJECTION — SHORT TERM TISSUE PRESERVATION AT 5°C.

1910 PHENOMENON OF ENHANCEMENT — TECHNIQUE FOR RENAL TRANSPLANTATION (CARREL)

"RACE" OF HOST IMPORTANT IN TRANSPLANTATION

1900 ABO BLOOD GROUPS

Frontispiece. The chronology of some major discoveries and concepts in transplantation.

THE

IMMUNOBIOLOGY
OF
TRANSPLANTATION

RUPERT BILLINGHAM

WILLYS SILVERS

University of Pennsylvania School of Medicine

PRENTICE-HALL, INC., *Englewood Cliffs, N. J.*

Current printing (last digit):

10 9 8 7 6 5 4 3 2 1

C—13-451682-6
P—13-451674-5

Library of Congress Catalog Card Number: 70-152444

PRINTED IN THE UNITED STATES OF AMERICA

PRENTICE-HALL INTERNATIONAL, INC., *London*
PRENTICE-HALL OF AUSTRALIA, PTY. LTD., *Sydney*
PRENTICE-HALL OF CANADA, LTD., *Toronto*
PRENTICE-HALL OF INDIA PRIVATE LIMITED, *New Delhi*
PRENTICE-HALL OF JAPAN, INC., *Tokyo*

To

ELIZABETH RUSSELL and P. B. MEDAWAR,
who initiated us into the field of transplantation biology,
and to all those who have grafted with us.

Foundations of Immunology Series

This series of monographs is intended to provide readers of diverse backgrounds with an authoritative and clear statement concerning significant aspects of immunology. Each volume represents an individual contribution by a distinguished scientist. As a series, they provide a comprehensive view of the field.

The editors have encouraged the individuality of each author in content and method of presentation. They have sought as the major objective of the series, that each monograph be comprehensible and of interest to a broad audience. The authors provide an authoritative treatment of important problems in major research areas, in which rapid development of new information requires an integrated and reliable evaluation. The series should therefore prove valuable to advanced college students, graduate students, medical students and house staff, practitioners of medicine, laboratory scientists, and teachers.

ABRAHAM OSLER
LEON WEISS

Preface

Despite the tremendous burgeoning of interest in the immunobiology of transplantation which has taken place over the decade, and the vast literature on the subject being laid down in scientific journals, reviews, and symposium volumes, there have been few attempts to present a general introductory account of the basic principles and general concepts of the subject and their origins, its unsolved problems, and its future prospects.

We have tried to achieve this goal for the benefit of advanced students and clinicians interested in the biological bases of the "uniqueness of the individual" and in the nature of the processes that have had to be thwarted in order to launch the new era of replacement surgery. We hope this book will enable the genetically, the surgically, and the immunologically unsophisticated reader to get a good insight into the subject commonly known as "transplantation," its methodology, and its own distinctive language, without overburdening him with unnecessary detail.

Limitations of space and the desire to produce an easily readable text precluded crediting many investigators whose contributions we have described and synthesized. To them we tender our apologies and beg their indulgence. We hope that the selected bibliographies at the end of each chapter will provide the means for readers to identify the unsung heroes of the plot and follow their contributions in extenso.

We are deeply indebted to our colleagues for helpful criticism and suggestions, to Mrs. Jean M. Billingham for the illustrations, and to Mrs. Marilee Heffron and Mrs. Martha Lubaroff for help with the manuscript.

It is a pleasure to acknowledge that our own research efforts and the gathering of the material for this book have been made possible largely by grants from the United States Public Health Service.

The Medical School
University of Pennsylvania

RUPERT BILLINGHAM
WILLYS SILVERS

Contents

Introduction

For centuries surgeons have yearned for the day, now close at hand, when it would be possible for them to replace damaged or diseased tissues or organs by grafts from other human beings or, perhaps more ambitiously, from other mammals, as a standard therapeutic procedure.

Since the beginning of this century biologists from a wide variety of disciplines, including experimental oncology, embryology, genetics, and endocrinology, have been making use of transplantation as a powerful analytic tool in the analysis of a wide range of problems. Indeed, a considerable body of workers have found that elucidation of the requirements of grafts for conservation of viability and normal functional activity, and devising means of meeting these, to be interesting and worthwhile research goals in themselves.

The transplantation of living cells, tissues, or organs for experimental or therapeutic purposes entails problems of two entirely different categories. The first is concerned directly with the act of transplantation itself. Mainly of a technological nature, these problems are associated with the procurement, preparation, temporary or long-term storage or "banking," and finally relocation of the grafts in such a manner that the normal healing processes, following appropriate surgical procedures where necessary, such as vascular anastomoses, suffice to ensure their survival and conservation of essential structure and function. In experimental animals and in man, the feasibility of replacement by grafting of blood, bone marrow, corneas, extensive areas of skin, kidneys, hearts, lungs, liver, small bowel, pancreas, and other endocrine tissues is firmly established. This indicates that adequate if not completely satisfactory solutions to these problems have been developed for the tissues and organs listed. For completeness, it is worth mentioning that the slow rate and inefficiency of nerve regeneration remain very serious obstacles that must be overcome before limb transplantation can be regarded as a worthwhile endeavor for the clinician.

The second category of problems is much more formidable and stems from the unrelenting incompatibility of *homografts* (i.e., grafts transplanted from one individual to another of the *same* species—also referred to as *allogeneic* grafts or *allografts*).

Homografts normally fail where *autografts* (grafts of which the donor is also the recipient) or *isografts* (sometimes referred to as syngeneic grafts; grafts of which the donor and recipient are of the *same* genetic constitution, as in the case of identical twins or members of the same inbred strain) transplanted in exactly the same manner are permanently successful. For example, if free skin autografts and homografts are placed on a common bed on the side of a rabbit's trunk, the autografts undergo a phase of minor reparative changes, including transient epidermal hyperplasia, and then reassume their original condition with a high degree of perfection. The homografts also heal in, acquire a rich blood supply, and behave as autografts do at first. Soon, however, they become inflamed and edematous and their dermis is heavily infiltrated by leucocytes, predominantly by lymphocytes and histiocytes. Cessation of blood flow, lymphatic drainage, and disruption of vessel walls, accompanied by the disintegration and separation of the entire epidermis and death of the cellular population of the graft, including the immigrant cells of host origin, soon follow. Finally, the necrotic graft is totally transformed into a desiccated, discolored scab which sloughs as a consequence of its being undermined by ingrowth of native host epidermis. This process of destruction, known as the *homograft reaction,* is usually complete within two weeks.

An essentially similar fate overtakes homografts of all other solid tissues (normal or malignant) or organs that establish vascular connections with their hosts of their own accord, or have them established surgically by vascular anastomoses. Of course, different symptoms are associated with the destruction process as it affects different kinds of homografts in different species. There is cessation of urine output in the case of the kidney homograft, altered electrical activity followed by diminishing output in the case of cardiac transplants, bilirubinemia and other biochemical changes in the constitution of the blood in the case of livers, and tumor homografts wane in size and eventually disappear. Cartilage loses its ability to take up radioactive sulfate ions, and ovarian homografts, in ovariectomized hosts, can no longer sustain sexual cycles. Thyroid grafts lose their power to take up radioactive iodine, and parathyroid grafts fail to maintain normal calcium levels in the blood of hosts whose own organs have been removed. Bone marrow grafts cease to contribute red cells of donor antigenic type to the blood stream, and the death of transplanted antibody-forming cells is indicated by the fall in titre of antibody of "adoptive" origin in their hosts. Another useful method for following the rejection of transplanted lymphoid cells entails labeling the cells before transfer with tritiated thymidine or chromium[51] and then following the elimination of these labels.

As we shall see, destruction of homografts is one of the most striking and reproducible of all immunological phenomena, manifested by all species of vertebrates so far tested. It is the outcome of a highly developed capacity of animals to recognize and treat as foreign and unwanted, cells from genetically dissimilar donors—a consequence of a cell surface allotypy determined by an extremely subtle and complex genetic polymorphism, the biological significance of which has yet to be elucidated.

Although the central core of transplantation immunology still comprises the classical themes of the genetic determination of homograft incompatibility and the nature of the processes which put it into effect, the subject embraces many additional facets and subdivisions which have arisen in large part from chance observations and their interpretation.

For example, Dr. Ray D. Owen's brilliant recognition and interpretation of the phenomenon of red cell chimerism in dizygotic twin cattle in 1945 prepared the way for the discovery of the principle of immunological tolerance in 1953, the basic principles of which were worked out, at least in broad outline, by means of the homograft immunity system. Studies with X rays, certain steroids, and other agents had indicated the feasibility of weakening the homograft reaction nonspecifically, thus initiating the field of immunosuppression on a systematic basis. However, work on immunological tolerance indicated that a *complete* solution to the homograft problem was attainable, at least at the laboratory level. Apart from its impact upon immunology, this work recruited many additional workers, including surgeons, to transplantation immunology.

Another important and largely accidental discovery was that grafts which contained significant numbers of lymphoid cells could, in experimentally definable situations, mount destructive reactions against their alien hosts, i.e., so-called *graft-versus-host* (GVH) reactions. Apart from uttering a caveat concerning possible dangers associated with the use of grafts of the lymphohematopoietic tissue system for therapeutic purposes, GVH reactions have afforded the basis of important, highly discriminatory, and quantitative "tools" in transplantation immunology. They have provided simple assays for immunologically competent cells, revealing their presence as normal components of the cell populations of blood, peritoneal exudates, and thoracic duct lymph. They have also shed a great deal of light upon the sequence of cytological events responsible for the destruction of homografts in conventional host-versus-graft reactions.

It is also worth mentioning that not only have the procedures of transplantation played an indispensable role in the elucidation of the functional significance of the thymus and the bursa of Fabricius, but also the homograft reaction has proved to be one of the most important immunological responses with which to evaluate their role.

The success which has attended deliberate attempts to devise effective means of tissue typing and to characterize at least the macromolecular carriers of the specificities involved (i.e., the chemistry of transplantation antigens) has been dramatic. It has drawn into the field workers whose prime interests are genetic polymorphisms, the relation of genes to their specific products, as well as membrane physiologists, since these products are evidently integrated components of cell membranes.

Also relevant to an understanding of the tremendous increase in popularity, effort, and accomplishment in the field of transplantation which has occurred in little more than a decade are the important two-way exchange of information and ideas between the laboratory and the clinic and the increasing tendency of biologists and surgeons to work together in either location. It is alleged that Pasteur once said that every surgical operation represented an experiment in bacteriology—happily this is no longer true. What *is* true is that, despite the degree of success that now attends renal transplantation, and to some extent that of liver and cardiac transplants in man, every clinical organ transplantation still represents an "experiment" in transplantation immunology.

Important discoveries can still be made and problems investigated in transplantation biology by procedures which, though sometimes demanding in terms of manual dexterity on the part of the investigator (as, for example, kidney, heart, or liver transplantation in rats) and in the genetic constitution of the experimental subjects, are very inexacting in terms of expensive equipment. Elaborate equipment and complex techniques are admittedly indispensable for the detailed elucidation of many problems and phenomena in transplantation immunology, such as the biochemistry of the antigens involved or quantitation of homograft reactivity at the cellular level in vitro. Yet the assertion which Simonsen made a few years ago that "in the whole field of modern transplantation biology there are few significant contributions which were not made with techniques of utter simplicity" still holds good.

As we shall see, transplantation biology is rich in those "exceptions" which Bateson adjured us to treasure. When there are none, he said, "the work gets so dull that no one cares to carry it further." Notable among these exceptions, and one that is currently receiving a great deal of attention, is the mammalian fetus which in outbred populations represents a homograft intimately united to the tissues of a mother who, in theory, would confidently have been expected to reject it.

One of the most successful and widely employed therapeutic homografts is the blood transfusion. The practicality of injecting fluids into veins was demonstrated by the famous British architect, Sir Christopher

Wren, in 1657. Within the next few years both indirect and direct transfusions of blood were performed in dogs. The first really successful clinical blood transfusion was performed in 1829 by a Guy's Hospital physician and obstetrician, James Blundell, on a patient suffering from postpartum hemorrhage. Sporadic transfusions were performed after this, the procedure being complicated by problems of coagulation and unrecognized incompatibility. The existence of blood groups in man was revealed by Karl Landsteiner in 1900. By about 1920 clinical transfusion was becoming fairly commonplace, though for a long time it remained an individual operation—a single donor, usually a relative, being chosen for each patient. Largely under the impetus of World War II, blood banks were instituted in the early 1940s when transfusion became a commonplace procedure. The discovery of the Rh blood group system in 1940, and recognition that it was responsible for erythroblastosis fetalis, initiated clinical interest in the immunobiology of the maternal-fetal relationship.

The flourishing and highly important discipline of tumor immunology has a history which is almost inextricable from that of the immunology of normal tissue grafts. It had an abortive beginning at the turn of the century. Nearly all the early workers labored under the delusion that they were studying cancer when they were, in fact, using tumors to study transplantation. As Woglom put it in 1929, "the tumor problem . . . was a tissue problem, resistance being directed against the tumor graft *as a strange tissue merely,* and not connected with any neoplastic qualities which the graft happened to possess."

Not until the immunogenetic principles of transplantation biology had been firmly established, properly inbred strains of mice had become available, and the need to study tumors of very recent origin was recognized, was the setting conducive for a fruitful reconsideration of the immunology of cancer. Following Foley's classic work in 1953, application of the techniques devised to study immunity to homografts revealed that the cells of tumors induced by chemicals, by some viruses, and other agents differ qualitatively from normal cells by antigens at their surfaces which behave like weak transplantation antigens and are capable of inciting immune responses.

One of the most exciting developments in transplantation immunology has resulted from the reinvestigation of heterologous *antilymphocyte serum,* or ALS, pioneered by the work of Woodruff and Anderson in 1963. Apart from its remarkable capacity to abrogate homograft reactions and other so-called cellular immunities, this relatively harmless biological agent has also been found to be highly effective in overcoming reactivity to *heterografts* (i.e., grafts of which donor and recipient belong to *different* species), enabling human skin, for example, to thrive on mice for many weeks. Previously little attention had been focused on the immunology of heterografts because of their exceedingly short life spans. With most species combinations they rarely healed in properly and barely displayed any functional activity at all. With a few exceptions, immunosuppressive procedures which were highly effective in extending the lives of homografts proved to be only marginally effective with heterografts. Thanks to ALS, interest in heterografts has recently been revived. Sir Peter Medawar pointed out recently that greater success is now being obtained with grafts *between* species than was obtained within species fifteen years ago. Guarded optimism now prevails that "zoografting" may eventually afford a solution to the increasingly acute logistic problem of donor organ procurement.

One thing that the pioneers of transplantation could not have envisaged was the tremendous influence their field was destined to exert upon immunology in general. Like the early students of delayed hypersensitivity to microorganisms and other agents, the early transplanters owed very little to "orthodox" immunologists who listened to their communications with bored politeness and often wondered whether the homograft reaction had anything to do with immunology at all. The only advice they gave was always directed toward further attempts to reveal the humoral antibodies which, ex cathedra, they felt must be the agents of graft destruction. Inability of dead cells to elicit sensitivity was just another shortcoming that encouraged some of them to believe that the homograft reaction was a phenomenon *sui generis.*

The chapters that follow describe the discovery of the principles of immunological enhancement and of immunological tolerance, the demonstration that immunologically competent cells are *normal* ingredients of the blood, the revelation of the functional significance of the thymus and, most recently, the discovery of the potency of ALS as an immunosuppressant. These are only a few of the contributions of transplantation biologists, or results of the application of their procedures, which have played a major role in revitalizing immunology. Especially important are the attention and effort which transplanters have drawn to the underdeveloped and neglected areas of immunology, notably the so-called "cellular immunities" to which the homograft reaction is so closely related.

REFERENCES

Billingham, R. E. 1966. Tissue transplantation: scope and prospect. Science 153:266–270.

Billingham, R. E. 1970. The origins and objectives of transplantation, p.1–21. *In* J. M. Anderson [ed.] The biology and surgery of tissue transplantation. Blackwell, Oxford, England.

Converse, J. M., and P. R. Casson. 1968. The historical background of transplantation, p. 3–10. *In* F. T. Rapaport and J. Dausset [ed.] Human transplantation. Grune and Stratton, New York.

Medawar, P. B. 1958. The immunology of transplantation, p. 144–176. *In* The Harvey lectures, 1956–1957. Academic Press, New York.

Medawar, P. B. 1958. The homograft reaction. Roy. Soc. (London), Proc., B. 148:145–166.

Moore, F. D. 1964. Give and take. The development of tissue transplantation. W. B. Saunders Co., Philadelphia.

Chapter 1

The Genetic Determination of the Fate of Grafts

"By and large, . . . the homograft-reaction intrudes into genetics at every level. . . ."—P. B. MEDAWAR, 1958.

Although tissue transplantation affords a common meeting ground or useful technical procedure for investigations in many different disciplines which include immunology, surgery, biochemistry, pathology, endocrinology, and reproductive biology, the field to which it is most closely related is genetics. The intimate relationship between these two subjects stems, of course, from the fact that the antigens which are responsible for evoking the *homograft reaction* are genetically determined, i.e., homograft rejection is an immunogenetic phenomenon.

The immunogenetics of transplantation has developed from the pursuit of two quite separate scientific objectives: (1) the study of grafts of tumors, motivated by the hope of developing an immunotherapeutic approach to malignant disease and (2) the clinical and experimental study of grafts of normal tissues oriented toward the goal of clinical replacement therapy of tissues and organs by grafting.

The first field of research originated in the work of the Danish biologist, C. O. Jensen, who discovered that tumors of spontaneous origin in mice could sometimes be propagated by grafting *living* cells from one mouse to another. In 1903 he reported that one such lineage of tumor cells had been passaged through nineteen hosts over a period of nineteen months. Jensen recognized that mice of different "races" were not all equally susceptible to the growth of the tumors he was studying, and he actually spoke of an "active immunity" in the more refractory animals.

In extensions of Jensen's work, other investigators found that different tumors varied considerably in the ease with which they could be propagated by grafting. Any one particular tumor displayed completely unpredictable ups and downs in its readiness to grow in an alien milieu. The general rule was that the tumor first grew and then regressed and disappeared after transplantation to an unrelated animal. Sometimes the tumor cell grafts appeared not to grow at all. Furthermore, a mouse in which a tumor had first become transiently established and then regressed failed to support even the temporary growth of the tumor if it was transplanted for a second time, though the host might or might not sustain the growth of other tumors of different origins. General agreement was soon reached that regression of these transplanted tumors was due to some kind of *active* "repudiation" of the graft by its host, rather than to death of the grafted cells as a result of inanition as Ehrlich had believed. Many early attempts were made to demonstrate that what appeared to be an "immunity" to transplanted tumors was of the same kind as that which was already known to be provoked by injection of microorganisms or foreign proteins, but in vain.

It was generally recognized that tumors differed from one another in their ease of transplantation, and it was appreciated that the "race" of the animal into which the tumor was grafted had a great deal to do with whether or not it would grow. However, it must be pointed out that in these early days of mammalian genetics, animals of the same "race" usually had little more in common than color, geographic origin, or family pedigree.

In 1902 and 1903 Leo Loeb showed that tumors originating in a partially inbred strain of Japanese waltzing mice nearly always grew progressively if transplanted to further Japanese waltzing mice, yet failed to grow in an unrelated stock of animals. This observation furnished a striking demonstration of a clear-cut and uniform difference in susceptibility between the two strains. Stimulated by this work, Tyzzer, in 1909, carried out some carefully controlled experiments which, together with their results, are summarized in Table 1.1. He found that F_1 hybrid mice produced by mating waltzing mice with mice of a resistant stock were always susceptible to the growth of the tumor. This suggested that the responsible

Table 1.1

Summarizing the results obtained by Tyzzer when he transplanted a mammary gland adenocarcinoma originating in Japanese waltzing mice into Japanese waltzing mice, unrelated "common" mice, and their F_1 and F_2 hybrids.

Host mice	*Number challenged with tumor*	*Number in which tumor grew*	*Number in which tumor regressed*
Japanese waltzing mice	145	142	3
Common mice	48	0	48
F_1 hybrids	70	69	1
F_2 hybrids	54	0	54

factors were determined by genes which expressed themselves in the heterozygous condition. Mice of the F_2 generation, derived from interbreeding F_1 animals, were resistant to tumor growth.

These results were exceedingly difficult to interpret at the time since they did not appear to fit any simple explanation of inheritance based on Mendel's theory. The fact that *all* the F_1 mice were susceptible suggested that tumor growth depended upon the presence of a dominant character. However, according to Mendelian principles, if susceptibility to tumor growth depended upon the expression of a single dominant gene, three-quarters of the F_2 population would be expected to be susceptible. The problem was resolved by Dr. C. C. Little in 1914. He proposed that acceptance of a tumor graft depended upon the graft tissue and the host possessing a *large* number of "susceptibility factors" in common, and that *each* of these was determined by independent genes. If the combination of factors present in the tumor graft did not match those possessed by the host animal, the tumor would not grow progressively.

The acceptance of tumor grafts from *both* inbred parental strains by F_1 hybrids followed from the fact that these inherit *one* complete set of chromosomes, including all the susceptibility genes, or *histocompatibility genes* as they are now known, from each parent. However, when F_1 animals are mated to one another, there is a random distribution to the gametes of different combinations of maternal and paternal chromosomes. The F_2 offspring are therefore genetically heterogeneous, bearing all possible combinations of the histocompatibility genes present in the two original parental strains. Thus only a proportion of them will, by chance, receive all the histocompatibility-determining factors present in one or the other parental strains and, consequently, accept grafts from that particular strain. More important, this proportion is predictable, depending on the number of histocompatibility genes by which the parental strains differ from each other.

For example, if the parental strains differ by a *single* gene, one strain being A/A and the other A′/A′ (see Fig. 1.1), then out of the four possible combinations into which the original pairs of genes can be reassorted in the F_2 progeny, half will bear the codominant susceptibility genes of both parental stocks (i.e., will be heterozygous A/A′), and one-quarter each will be homozygous for one histocompatibility gene or the other (A/A or A′/A′). Consequently 75% of the offspring would be expected to accept grafts from either parental strain, though it may be noted that an animal which accepted a graft from one parental strain would not necessarily accept a graft from the other parental strain as well.

If the parental strains differ by two histocompatibility genes, i.e., two genetic loci are involved, then it can be shown that 56% ($^9/_{16}$) of their F_2 offspring should accept grafts from one of the parental strains. This is

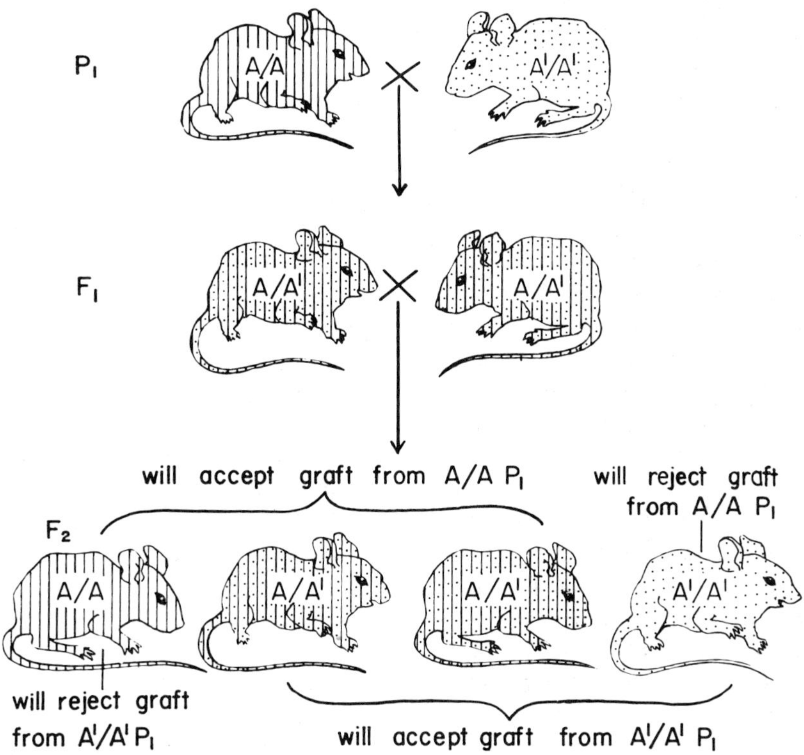

Fig. 1.1. If parental strain (P_1) animals differ at only a single histocompatibility locus, one being of genotype A/A and the other of genotype A′/A′, then four possible genetic combinations, two of which produce similar offspring, can occur in animals of the second generation (F_2). Thus, three out of four animals of the F_2 generation will possess at least one specific histocompatibility gene from one of the P_1 grandparents and, consequently, will tolerate a skin graft taken from any member of the inbred strain to which that grandparent happens to belong. One of four members of the F_2 population will reject grafts from this strain since it has not received a histocompatibility allele from it. The same situation holds true for grafts taken from the other P_1 strain. Regardless of the number of genes by which any P_1 pair differs, all first-generation (F_1) offspring will accept a graft donated by a member of either P_1 inbred strains.

true provided, of course, that each histocompatibility locus is inherited independently, i.e., the two loci are not linked. Furthermore, it can be shown that, in the F_2 population derived from any given pair of *inbred* strains, the proportion of animals susceptible to growth of a parental strain tumor will be equal to $(3/4)^n$, where the exponential, n, is simply the number of histocompatibility loci at which the parental strains differ.

Little and Tyzzer set out to test this idea in 1916. They outcrossed Japanese waltzing mice with an unrelated inbred strain to produce a large F_2 population, each member of which was challenged with carcinoma tissue of Japanese waltzer origin. Only three of the 183 hosts (1.6%) accepted their grafts. This percentage was consistent with a value for *n* of about 14 or 15, indicating that the original mouse strains differed by about 14 or 15 histocompatibility factors.

Another method of determining the number of histocompatibility genes in respect of which a tumor-susceptible and a tumor-resistant strain of mice differ involves mating their F_1 hybrids with mice of the tumor-resistant parental strain to produce R_2 backcross animals. In this case it can be shown that the proportion of R_2 mice susceptible to the tumor will be $(\frac{1}{2})^n$ where *n* is the number of histocompatibility loci with respect to which the parental strains differ.

While further details of the genetics of tumor transplantation were being worked out by Dr. G. D. Snell, Little's successor, and his associates at the Jackson Laboratory at Bar Harbor, Maine, Dr. Peter Gorer, a pathologist at Guy's Hospital, London, was engaged in classic studies destined to help bridge the existing wide gap between knowledge of the genetic determination of histoincompatibility and the manner of its fulfillment. In 1938 Gorer demonstrated by serologic means the existence of antigenic variation among the red cells of mice and, more important, that one antigen, which he designated as "antigen II" was common to red cells, normal tissue cells, and tumor cells of one particular strain. Confrontation of mice lacking this antigen with sarcoma grafts from donors possessing this antigen resulted in regression of the tumor graft and excited the formation of an isoantibody directed against it. On the basis of these and other findings, Gorer reformulated Little's genetical theory of transplantation in immunological terms as follows:

> *"Normal and neoplastic tissues contain isoantigenic factors which are genetically determined. Isoantigenic factors present in the grafted tissue and absent in the host are capable of eliciting a response which results in destruction of the graft. Under special circumstances, the response may not be elicited or the graft may not be destroyed thereby."*

Gorer's own early work afforded almost decisive evidence that resistance to the growth of transplanted tumors and, by implication, that of normal tissue grafts, is an immunological phenomenon. However, as he realized, the isoantibodies he had discovered were not necessarily the effectors of graft destruction.

The second field of research which has made major contributions to the immunogenetics of transplantation is that concerned with the grafting of *normal* tissues. It had its own independent origins and history and for many years there was little interchange between those who worked with tumors and those interested in the use of transplantation for clinical replacement purposes. With a few notable but unheeded exceptions, the pioneers of plastic surgery usually failed to make any distinction between skin grafts of autologous and those of homologous origin.

Bauer's finding, in 1927, that skin grafts exchanged between identical twins in man are permanently accepted was consistent with the thesis that compatibility of normal tissue grafts, like that of tumor grafts, is genetically determined.

The first important landmark in the study of homografts of *normal* tissues was Gibson and Medawar's critical study of the fates of autografts and of "first-set" and subsequent, or "second-set" skin homografts (grafts originating from the *same* donor) on a patient in Scotland in 1943. This work was closely followed by Medawar's classic analyses of the fate of skin homografts in rabbits which established both the basic pathophysiology of the homograft reaction and its immunologic nature.

Among the various lines of evidence he obtained in support of the thesis that the rejection of skin homografts is an immunological phenomenon are the following:

1. Resistance to skin homografts is not innate; homografts transplanted to hitherto ungrafted hosts enjoy a brief latent period of apparent well-being during which their cells may proliferate freely.

2. There is a definite though weak dosage effect, tiny homografts having a longer expectation of survival than larger ones, though the dose-response curve is very flat.

3. Once called into being, the sensitivity evoked by homografts is *systemic,* i.e., generalized throughout all parts of the body supplied by blood vessels.

4. The existence of a state of homograft immunity is revealed in terms of the accelerated or peremptory manner in which "second-set" homografts are destroyed. Initially this was interpreted as the homologue of the "secondary response" of the immunologist.

5. The homograft reaction is highly specific. For example, a rabbit R, which has received and rejected skin homografts from a donor D_1, will reject subsequent grafts of D_1's skin in an accelerated manner (the "second-set" response), yet will usually treat skin homografts from an unrelated, third-party donor, D_2, as if they are first-set grafts.

Medawar's early work also focused attention upon the many advantages of skin over all other tissues—normal or malignant—for quantitative studies on the homograft reaction. Most important of these is the measure of the intensity of the host's response afforded by the fairly easily determined *survival time* of a graft. Grafts can be judged alive or dead by histological examination of biopsy specimens or, with a little experience, on the basis of macroscopic examination with a fair degree of accuracy.

From assessments of the individual survival times of the homografts borne by a panel of hosts, a useful statistic, the *median survival time* (MST) of the homografts can be determined in much the same way as median lethal doses are arrived at in pharmacology. The MST represents the time at which the last surviving remnants of epithelium of the skin homografts carried by 50% of the subjects have just broken down.

Validity for the belief that conclusions drawn from studies on skin homografts were applicable to homografts of other tissues was furnished by Dr. W. J. Dempster of the Postgraduate Medical School of London and Dr. Morton Simonsen of Copenhagen. Working independently in the early 1950s, these investigators initiated carefully controlled studies on renal homografts in dogs, using surgical procedures developed by Alexis Carrel at the beginning of the century.

From the various studies described above, the general principles of transplantation immunogenetics emerged which may be formulated as follows:

1. Acceptance or rejection of a graft is determined by the presence or absence of alien, genetically determined antigens in the grafted cells, known as *transplantation antigens.* The genes responsible for the formation of these cellular antigens are known as *histocompatibility genes,* and the chromosomal locations of these genes are *histocompatibility* loci, or *H* loci. At each of these loci a series or family of alternative genes, or *alleles,* may occur.

2. Histocompatibilty alleles are codominant, i.e., their end products are individually demonstrable in the heterozygote (as, for example, with the A and B blood group alleles in man where both antigens A and B occur on heterozygous AB erythrocytes). Thus isografts (or syngeneic grafts)—grafts between individuals of the *same* genetic constitution, for instance, identical twins or members of the same *isogenic strain* *—are always accepted.

3. Grafts from isogenic parental strain animals to their F_1 hybrids are also permanently accepted, as Little and Tyzzer had previously found, since the F_1 hybrid possesses all the antigens of both its parental strains.

4. Grafts from F_1 hybrids are promptly rejected by animals of either parental strain since they confront each strain with one set of antigens characteristic of the other strain.

---

* A strain is designated "isogenic" or "syngeneic" when there have been twenty or more consecutive generations of brother × sister matings, or twenty or more consecutive generations of parent-offspring matings, provided that the offspring was mated to the younger parent. As a result of this inbreeding procedure, all the animals of a particular strain are homozygous at all, or virtually all, loci; hence, their progeny receive representatives of *all* the histocompatibility genes that characterize the strain.

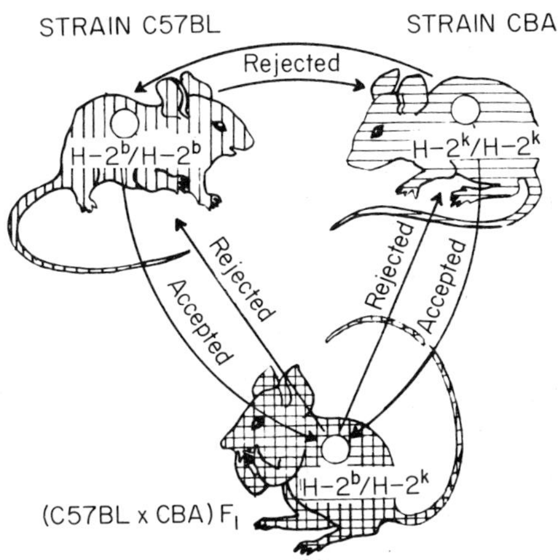

Fig. 1.2. Fates of skin homografts exchanged between mice of two different inbred strains, C57BL and CBA, and their F_1 hybrid. Although only the histocompatibility-2 genotypes of the two strains are represented in the diagram, it should be borne in mind that they differ at a multiplicity of histocompatibility loci, each of which behaves similarly. Since histocompatibility alleles are codominant, the F_1 hybrid possesses *all* of the transplantation antigens present in both parental strains. Only those homografts are accepted which have no antigens that are not also represented in the host.

These simple principles are illustrated in Fig. 1.2.

Because of the development of increasing numbers of different inbred strains of mice from about 1920 onward, a tremendous amount of information has accumulated concerning the genetics of histocompatibility in this species. However, the progressive development and/or availability of inbred strains of other species, including guinea pigs, rats, hamsters, chickens, and platyfish, has enabled the scope of transplantation immunogenetics to be greatly expanded in recent years. As we shall see later, another recent factor which has expedited progress in this field has been the development of serologic and other procedures for studying transplantation antigens in members of outbred populations such as man.

From the immunologic viewpoint, the F_2 test affords a crude estimate of the number of transplantation antigens with respect to which the members of two given inbred strains differ and against which they can react immunologically. To the geneticist the F_2 test can provide only a *minimal* estimate of the number of different histocompatibility loci present in a given species. This follows from the fact that, if the particular strains tested happen to carry the *same* allele at any locus, this locus will make no contribution to the estimate of the gene (or locus) number. Furthermore, it is known that some types of grafts fail to detect loci which are demonstrable with other types of tissue graft. For example, it is well known that tumor grafts are frequently accepted despite their possession of some antigens that are foreign to the host, i.e., the growth potential of many tumors is such that it seems to enable them to override any minor histoincompatibilities which prevail. A similar situation occurs with grafts of some endocrine tissues (see Chapter 6). Skin homografts appear to be the most exacting of all tissues insofar as their genetic requirements for acceptance are concerned. Being highly susceptible to weak levels of immunity, skin homografts are the ones of choice for discriminating definitions of histocompatibility relationships.

Finally, since linkage between certain histocompatibility loci has been shown to occur in mice, and more such relationships will undoubtedly be discovered in this and other species, it is obvious that a single locus, as defined by the F_2 or R_2 tests may, in certain instances, eventually prove to comprise two or more closely linked genes.

Number of Histocompatibility Loci in Different Species

Despite its limitations, the F_2 test has provided some insight into the number of histocompatibility loci present in different species.

In mice and rats, applications of the test to some of the different strain combinations available have indicated the existence of upwards of fifteen to seventeen loci (see Chapter 3). In guinea pigs, which have a very long history of domestication, only two inbred strains, #2 and #13, are available. These were developed by Dr. Sewall Wright about sixty years ago from a single laboratory population. Evidence of the existence of only about seven or eight loci has been obtained for these animals.

In Syrian hamsters not more than three loci are necessary to account for the rejection of skin grafts exchanged between the members of different strains. It is worth pointing out, however, that all domestic hamsters, including the inbred strains available, are descendants of a single male and two female littermates captured in Syria in 1930. Either the apparent paucity of histocompatibility loci in this species results from the "unitary" origin of the animals, or it may reflect the situation in wild hamster populations. Since recent skin grafting studies conducted on hamsters of a different subspecies caught in the wild revealed that a high degree of graft compatibility prevailed in them, the simple histocompatibility relationships in domesticated Syrian hamsters may indeed reflect the situation in nature.

In animals where only outbred populations are available, there is no way of obtaining an accurate estimate of the number of histocompatibility loci present. However, from a study involving the mutual exchange of grafts between twenty-two members of a heterogeneous population of rabbits, Medawar calculated that a minimal number of seven loci must exist in this species.* In man, from an analysis of the fate of skin homografts from multiple donors transplanted to a single recipient, Dr. William Longmire and his associates suggested a minimum number of twenty-three loci. From the wealth of clinical information available concerning the consistency with which homografts are rejected in man, whether from unrelated or from consanguineous donors, and from a limited amount of experimental evidence obtained from studies on volunteers, it seems safe to conclude that, so far as the number of our histocompatibility loci is concerned, we resemble mice and rats much more closely than we do hamsters.

Obviously the polymorphism which exists with respect to histocompatibility factors in a given population will depend upon (1) the number of loci and (2) the number of different alleles at each locus, and their relative frequencies. As we shall see, the latter factor is the more important and the existence of only a single locus with an extensive series of alleles with similar frequencies could account for a high incidence of incompatibility when grafts are exchanged between individuals selected at random or even when tissues are grafted between related individuals. In fact, an important locus of this kind does occur in mice and man and probably in other species as well.

For reasons already mentioned, the mouse has long been the animal of choice for detailed analyses of the genetic basis of histocompatibility. Consequently most of what follows will be concerned with work conducted in this species. However, as information has accumulated from genetic studies in other species, including man, it is becoming increasingly evident that the mouse has been an excellent prototype. Indeed, the similarities which have already been discovered between the genetics of tissue transplantation in mice and man are so striking as to make it seem doubtful whether many new principles will emerge as further information is obtained in the latter species.

Although studies on grafts made to F_2 and backcross generations provide evidence for the existence of multiple histocompatibility loci, they tell us nothing about the identity of the loci, nor do they permit any separation of the loci from one another. In the sections that follow methods will be described which have enabled the loci to be separated and analyzed.

---

* More recently Dr. C. K. Chai of the Jackson Laboratory has estimated that rabbits have at least 20 histocompatibility loci, and perhaps more than three times this number. His calculations were based on the percentage of surviving skin grafts in lines which had been brother × sister mated for from 5 to 17 generations.

Production and Utilization of Congenic Resistant Strains

Special stocks of animals, known as *congenic resistant* or *CR strains,* have played a virtually indispensable role in elucidation of the genetics of histocompatibility in mice. Some consideration of the manner in which these stocks are produced is necessary to understand fully the information which has been derived from them.

By alternately backcrossing and inbreeding to a particular reference stock, as illustrated in Fig. 1.3, populations of animals can be produced which are of essentially the same genotype except for a difference at *one* histocompatibility locus—the one which has been selected for. By carrying

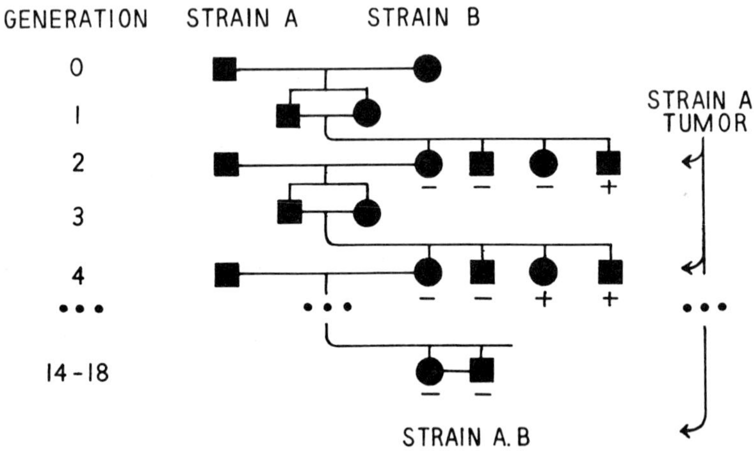

Fig. 1.3. Illustrating the method of producing congenic resistant lines of mice. In this pedigree chart, A is a mouse belonging to *any* isogenic strain, and B is a member of some other strain which need not be genetically uniform—indeed, it could be a trapped wild mouse. Animals A and B are mated, and an F_2 generation is raised. The animals of this generation and of all subsequent inbreeding generations (those which are even-numbered) are challenged with a test tumor of strain A origin. Survivors, animals that reject their tumor grafts (indicated by a minus sign), as opposed to those that succumb to them (indicated by a plus sign), are mated back, i.e., backcrossed, to strain A. After seven or eight such backcrosses, nearly all the alleles not closely linked with the histocompatibility factor that has been selected for will have been replaced by alleles from strain A. Consequently, in generations 14 or 16, two survivors (tumor-resistant mice) may be mated together to produce a congenic resistant strain, A.B. The latter carries one histocompatibility gene derived from strain B which differs from the corresponding or allelic gene in strain A. Apart from this difference, strain A.B has essentially the same genetic constitution as A and, accordingly, is designated as a *congenic resistant or CR line.* Of course, because of this difference at a single histocompatibility locus, grafts exchanged in either direction between A and A.B will carry a foreign transplantation antigen and will be rejected. (From Snell, G.D. 1958. J. Nat. Cancer Inst. 21:843.)

out specific breeding tests with these strains and by challenging the offspring produced with tumors of known genotype, it has been possible to identify different histocompatibility loci and to assign to each of them two or more alleles.

Once a group of CR lines on one or more genetic backgrounds has been established, the problem remains of identifying the particular histocompatibility locus as well as the specific allele selected for. Obviously two CR lines from the same initial cross may be different or they may be identical. The process by which each is produced merely selects at *random* an alien allele at *some* histocompatibility locus for introduction onto the chosen genetic background. There are two methods for analyzing CR lines:

1. *Analysis by the F_1 Test.* To determine whether two lines, congenic with strain A and therefore resistant to a strain A tumor graft, are congenic for histocompatibility alleles at *different* loci, they are mated and their F_1 progeny challenged with the A strain tumor. If alleles at *different* loci are involved, the tumor will be accepted since the genotypes of the two congenic lines will complement each other, and their F_1 offspring will therefore possess *all* the histocompatibility genes present in A. If, however, the two strains are congenic for different alleles at the *same* locus, their F_1 hybrid would still differ at that particular locus from strain A and would therefore reject a tumor of A strain origin.* Whether the two CR lines bear the same or different alleles can be determined by exchanging skin grafts between them.

2. *Analysis by Linkage.* Because a large number of mouse mutations have been assigned to specific linkage groups, i.e., have been "mapped" (the mouse has twenty pairs of chromosomes), it has been possible to "map" a few histocompatibility loci. Linkage analysis for histocompatibility loci is facilitated when the parents of congenic lines happen to differ by genes with visible effects which are closely linked with histocompatibility genes. Such genes serve as "markers." The introduction of the histocompatibility gene onto the inbred background introduces the marker gene also and, in later intercross generations, the linkage becomes apparent through an association of the marker gene with resistance to a test graft.

One fortuitous example of this occurred when, in developing a con-

---

* It should be noted, however, that there are rare instances in which an F_1 hybrid of two congenic lines, each of which is congenic with respect to *different* alleles at the *same* locus, will accept a skin graft from a congenic stock bearing yet another allele at this locus. For example, (B10.D2 × B10.BR)F_1 mice will accept skin grafts from B10.A animals even though the B10.D2, B10.BR, and B10.A congenic lines all differ with regard to their H-2 genotype. This is due to the fact that the antigenic specificities determined by the H-2 alleles of B10.D2 and B10.BR mice include all of those determined by the H-2 allele of B10.A animals.

genic resistant line from an initial cross between a pigmented strain of mice, C57BL/10, and an albino strain, BALB/c, it was discovered that there was an association between a histocompatibility factor, subsequently designated as H-1, and albinism (which is determined by the so-called C locus). Further tests demonstrated that the H-1 and C loci were about seven units apart in linkage group I.

This linkage information is important because it provides another means of differentiating one locus from another. A histocompatibility locus which is assigned to a particular position on the linkage map must, of necessity, differ from a histocompatibility locus occupying another position on the map. Thus, when another histocompatibility locus was subsequently found to be associated with linkage group I, its distinction from H-1 could be confirmed by demonstrating that its relationship to the C locus differed considerably from that of H-1. This locus, which is about twenty-four units from H-1, was named H-4.

So far fifteen histocompatibility loci have actually been identified in the mouse. Of these, five autosomal loci (H-1, H-2, H-3, H-4, and H-13), a Y-linked locus, and an X-linked locus, have now been assigned to specific linkage groups.

Relative Strengths of Antigens Determined by Different Loci

The relative strengths of the antigens determined by these different loci have been evaluated by exchanging skin grafts between members of the appropriate congenic resistant lines. It was soon found that the barriers which the products of different loci oppose to transplantation differed widely. Accordingly we refer to "major" and "minor" loci, with corresponding "strong" and "weak" antigens. A difference between donor and host with respect to a single strong antigen (or allele at a major locus) is usually sufficient to elicit a homograft reaction of near maximal intensity, so that a skin graft is destroyed within about eleven days. On the other hand, a difference at a minor locus may enable a skin homograft to live in a state of apparent normality for upwards of one hundred days before it is eventually overcome by the host.

The H–2 Locus of the Mouse

Because one histocompatibility locus of the mouse, known as the H-2, seems to predominate above all others in terms of the potency of its products and its genetic complexity, and because an increasing weight of evidence suggests that the rat, man, chicken, and probably other species possess a locus with properties similar to H-2, a brief outline of our knowledge of this locus is essential.

We have already mentioned the pioneer work of Peter Gorer who demonstrated the sharing in common of an antigen, Antigen II, by tumor tissue and erythrocytes of mice of a particular strain. The gene locus determining this antigen, now known as H-2, was subsequetly shown, by virtue of its close linkage to a dominant gene, *Fu,* which causes fusion of tail vertebrae, to be in the ninth linkage group. The linkage of H-2 and *Fu* has proven to be very helpful since, just as linkage relationships can be employed to distinguish one locus from another, as was the case with H-1 and H-4, they can also be utilized to confirm allelism. Thus the linkage of H-2 with *Fu* and other genes in linkage group IX has been employed to demonstrate the existence of twenty alleles at the H-2 locus. Moreover, a recent survey conducted by P. Iványi of the H-2 genotypes of wild mice trapped in the city of Prague suggests that many more alleles must also occur at this locus. Indeed, a figure in the hundreds would not be at all surprising.

Much of our information concerning the H-2 locus has been forthcoming from serological studies. This work has been facilitated by the ease with which isoantibodies reactive with H-2 determined specificities on erythrocytes and other cells are produced and demonstrated. In contrast, antibodies reactive with the specificities determined by other histocompatibility loci are much more difficult to produce and/or demonstrate. Among the serological tests employed are hemagglutination, hemolysis, leukoagglutination, and cytotoxicity; the last uses lymphocytes as "target" cells.

When serological analyses were performed on cells of animals of different H-2 genotypes, the important discovery was made that there is a good deal of cross-reactivity between antisera prepared against supposedly different H-2 factors. This cross-reactivity was subsequently shown to be due to the presence of *multiple* specificities in each antiserum, some of which were directed against antigens shared in common by the products of two or more H-2 alleles. This suggested that the H-2 locus, like the Rh locus in man, is a complex locus comprised of a series of very closely linked genes, or *pseudoalleles,* each of which determines a single specificity and which are normally inherited *en bloc*. This concept received further support when crossing-over within the H-2 system was reported. The frequency of recombination between the components D and K, which are situated at different ends of the complex, is about 1%.

Most of our knowledge of the H-2 locus has come from the painstaking efforts of Dr. G. D. Snell and his "school." By using many different isogenic strains, as well as congenic resistant strains known to differ only with regard to their H-2 genotype, for the production of antisera which were then studied by absorption and cross-absorption procedures, these investigators have detected and identified more than thirty serologically distinct specificities on mouse erythrocytes. The majority of these are determined by the H-2 locus. Indeed, at the present time, it is believed that the various alleles at the H-2 locus are involved in determining no less than twenty-four different specificities * which collectively characterize the locus. Some of the known alleles and specificities of the H-2 system and the isogenic strains that carry them are presented in Table 1.2. As

Table 1.2

The H-2 alleles of some common inbred strains of mice and the antigenic specificities associated with them.

H-2 alleles	*Antigenic specificities*																			*Inbred strains in which alleles are present*
	1	*2*	*3*	*4*	*5*	*6*	*8*	*10*	*11*	*13*	*14*	*22*	*25*	*27*	*28*	*29*	*31*	*32*	*33*	
a	+		+	+	+	+	+	+	+	+	+		+	+	+	+				A, AKR.K
b		+			+	+					+	+		+	+	+			+	C57BL/6, 129
d			+	+		+	+	+		+	+			+	+	+	+			BALB/c, DBA/2
k	+		+		+		+		+				+					+		CBA, C3H, AKR

While only four alleles (a, b, d, and k) are represented here, upwards of twenty alleles, each determining a different battery of antigenic specificities, have been defined.

Specificities 7, 9, 16, 17, 19, and 30 are not included in this table because they are associated with one or more of the other alleles.

Note that there is considerable antigenic overlapping between the specificities determined by different alleles, and in no instance is any allele associated with more than fourteen specificities. (See text.)

this table shows, there is considerable antigenic overlapping between the specificities determined by the different alleles. Moreover, although the number of specificities determined by each allele is highly variable, in no instance does it exceed fourteen. It can easily be seen how this multiplicity of antigenic specificities can be rearranged, through crossing-over, to produce an almost unlimited number of possible H-2 alleles. Indeed, it seems apparent that almost every time a crossover occurs within the H-2 complex a different allele is formed.

Only relatively recently has attention been focused on the genetic systems responsible for histoincompatibility in other mammals, primarily in rats and man. The former species has attracted attention because of the increasing number of isogenic strains that have become available and the

* Thirty-three specificities have been assigned to this locus, but uncertainty remains concerning specificities 15, 20, 21, 23, and 24. Furthermore, recent evidence suggests that specificities 6, 18, 26, and 28 are determined by genes which, though in linkage group IX, are distinct from H-2.

extensive studies on tolerance, organ transplantation, and graft-versus-host reactivity conducted with rats. Man is under intensive study because of the tremendous interest in clinical transplantation and the desire to improve the prognosis of organ homotransplantation by tissue typing.

The situation in the rat parallels that in the mouse very closely not only in terms of the number of histocompatibility loci, as already mentioned, but also in that a single locus, the Ag-B (or H-1) locus, seems to exert a predominant influence on the fate of homografts and other manifestations of transplantation immunity. Its specificities are also detectable on red cells. Evidence is emerging that, like those of the H-2 locus of the mouse, the products of the Ag-B locus are also complexes comprising a larger number of individual specificities in different combinations. At present, twenty-one antigenic specificities have been attributed to this locus, but no more than ten of these have been found to be associated with any one allele. Alhough the number of alleles thus far recognized at the Ag-B locus is only nine, this is obviously a very minimal figure, due to the paucity of unrelated stocks available for testing.

While birds reject homografts as vigorously as mammals, and though chickens, ducks, and to a lesser extent other avian species have been used extensively in transplantation studies, our knowledge of their histocompatibility systems is not very great. The number of histocompatibility loci in chickens has recently been estimated to be of the order of nine to thirteen. However, this is almost certainly an underestimate since it is based on skin grafting birds of the first backcross generation produced from crosses involving only four different lines. Here again there appears to be one predominant histocompatibility locus, known as the B locus, which, like the H-2 locus of mice and the Ag-B locus of rats, is characterized by a series of multiple alleles each of which determines a battery of antigenic specificities. Moreover, this locus is also involved in the determination of red-cell antigens. The importance of this locus in transplantation reactions is indicated by the fact that the ability of homologous cellular inocula to produce graft-versus-host reactions (see Chapter 11) in embryonic chickens is dependent on the host possessing an antigen at the B locus which the graft does not have.

REFERENCES

Batchelor, J. R. 1965. Histocompatibility systems. Brit. Med. Bull. 21:100–105.

Elkins, W. L., and J. Palm. 1966. Identification of a single strong histocompatibility locus in the rat by normal spleen-cell transfer. Ann. N.Y. Acad. Sci. 129:573–580.

Lengerová, A. 1969. Immunogenetics of tissue transplantation. John Wiley & Sons, Inc., New York.

Little, C. C. 1956. The genetics of tumor transplantation, p. 279–309. *In* George D. Snell [ed.] Biology of the laboratory mouse. Dover Publications, Inc., New York.

Schierman, L. W., and A. W. Nordskog. 1962. Relationship of erythrocyte to leukocyte antigens in chickens. Science 137:620–621.

Snell, G. D., and J. H. Stimpfling. 1966. Genetics of tissue transplantation, p. 457–491. *In* E. L. Green [ed.] Biology of the laboratory mouse (2nd ed.). McGraw Hill, New York.

Śtark, O., B. Frenzl, and V. Kŕen. 1968. Erythrocyte and transplantation antigens in inbred strains of rats. Folia Biol. (Praha) 14:169–175.

Chapter 2

The Genetics of Histocompatibility in Man

In man there appear to be two major histocompatibility systems in addition to an unknown number of minor ones. The first is determined by the ABO blood group antigens and the second by a compound system of determinants known as the HL-A (formerly Hu-1) system (Human Leukocyte Antigen System). The latter bears a striking similarity to the H-2 locus of the mouse and the Ag-B locus of the rat.

ABO Antigens and Histocompatibility

Compatibility with regard to ABO antigens has long been recognized to be of paramount importance in the clinical "transplantation," or transfusion, of blood from the viewpoint of avoiding transfusion reactions.* However, only within the last five years has ABO compatibility been implicated as an important factor in the transplantation of other tissues and organs, notably skin and kidneys. Although it was recognized that kidneys transplanted across major ABO group barriers were particularly susceptible to a rapid and violent type of rejection, it was generally assumed that this was a consequence of the presence of "contaminating," incompatible donor red cells. Since, even after thorough perfusion of the donor organ, its vessels still contain significant numbers of donor erythrocytes and leucocytes (which also have ABO antigens), agglutination reactions directed against these cells might exert an *indirect* adverse effect on the survival of the organ as a whole. Indeed, this mechanism has still not been ruled out as playing a significant role in acute rejections of renal grafts. However, in the light of recent findings that ABO antigens on fixed tissue cells can

* Anti-A antibodies occur naturally in the plasma of persons whose cells lack this antigen, and anti-B antibodies occur in the plasma of persons whose cells do not contain B. The presence of these antibodies in the plasma of a recipient of a transfusion causes agglutination of donor erythrocytes if the latter carry the corresponding "incompatible" antigen.

behave like "conventional" transplantation antigens, their role in organ transplantation has had to be reconsidered.

Whereas in both mice and rats there is no convincing evidence that injection of hosts with pure (leucocyte-free) preparations of H-2 or Ag-B incompatible red cells, respectively (which do bear serologically detectable specificities corresponding to these loci), will elicit transplantation immunity, this is not the case with the A and B erythrocyte antigens in man.

Dausset and Rapaport found that, when group O human volunteers were injected with leukocyte-free AB erythrocytes and challenged two weeks later with skin grafts from *other* AB donors and from group O donors, the AB donor grafts were rejected in an accelerated or second-set manner, whereas the O grafts were rejected as primary or first-set homografts. Moreover, A and B substances, isolated from the gastric mucosae of hogs and horses, respectively, were equally effective in inducing sensitivity with respect to skin homografts. The failure of pure red cells from ABO-*compatible* donors to sensitize human hosts against skin homografts indicates that these cells do not possess effective amounts of other transplantation antigens.

Despite the importance of the ABO antigens in clinical transplantation, it has yet to be determined whether the immunological resistance they provoke is of the same kind as that evoked by the histocompatible antigens associated with the nucleate cells of solid tissues.

Leucocyte Antigens and Histocompatibility

The history of leucocyte grouping dates back to Medawar's demonstration in 1946 that the intradermal injection of leucocytes from a rabbit D into a rabbit R induced a state of sensitivity to subsequent grafts of D's skin. This established the important fact that leucocytes and skin and, as later work indicated, other organs such as kidneys share at least some important transplantation antigens in common. The subsequent observation that tolerance of skin homografts can be induced in very young rodents by inoculation with living leucocytes of the same alien genetic origin indicated that leucocytes must express *all* the transplantation antigens that a skin graft has and, by implication, other tissues and organs of the body as well (see Chapter 10). These findings, in conjunction with the ease with which leucocytes can be obtained, explain why leucocyte grouping is so important in histocompatibility testing.

Note that, insofar as all immunogenetic studies on man have to be carried out on heterogeneous populations, modifications of the procedures employed for inbred populations have had to be devised.

As a consequence of refinements of technique, leucocyte serology began to get under way in the early 1950s. Most of it was conducted on patients transfused repeatedly, who were often found to possess antibodies capable of reacting with leucocytes from certain other donors, but not with their *own* leucocytes. A not unexpected complication in this work was that the antibodies produced by individuals who had received repeated blood transfusions frequently "recognized" *many* different antigens, i.e., they were polyvalent. The availability of *monospecific* reagents is, of course, an essential prerequisite for grouping purposes.

The finding by Rose Payne in California and by J. J. Van Rood in Holland that pregnancy frequently leads to the formation of leucocyte antibodies in man not only solved the logistic problem of obtaining a good supply of sera containing leucocyte antibodies, but also helped to minimize the multiple specificity problem. This followed from the fact that, unlike a person who has received many transfusions, a woman who has been pregnant will only form antibodies against antigens carried by her husband and absent in her (provided that she hasn't received any blood transfusions). Thus these antibodies will be of limited specificity, sometimes being capable of identifying only a single antigen. Sera from human volunteers immunized by means of skin grafts or leucocytes are equally advantageous.

Selecting useful typing sera from the many sera available posed another problem. This was solved by the "computer approach" in which a large number of antisera are tested against a panel of one hundred or more leucocyte samples from different donors. The information obtained is analyzed with the aid of a computer to select sera reacting with identical or antithetical antigens. These sera are then investigated for monospecificity and tested in population and family studies. The exchange of typing sera among laboratories in different parts of the world and the holding of several international workshops in histocompatibility typing have played an indispensable role in defining the reagents and the antigens, arriving at a standard nomenclature, and indicating the high degree of consistency of the results obtainable.

By means of this approach more than twenty different leucocyte antigens have been recognized, most of them belonging to the HL-A system. From the information now available, this genetic system is visualized as an extended chromosomal segment possessing at least three subloci or mutational sites. More than thirty different HL-A alleles have so far been identified, and the finding of many more can confidently be anticipated. Moreover, by means of skin grafting experiments, five of the antigenic specificities determined by these alleles (more appropriately, *pseudoalleles*) have been identified as transplantation antigens.

The clinical importance of HL-A antigens is evident from the initial finding that skin grafts exchanged between siblings with identical HL-A type antigens survive significantly longer than grafts exchanged between unmatched sibling controls.

Unlike H-2 antigens, the specificities determined by the HL-A system have not, as yet, been shown to be present on red cells.

Since the antigens determined by the HL-A locus, as well as antigens belonging to a completely separate so-called group-5 system, are present on granulocytes, lymphocytes, platelets, and all tissues and organs thus far studied systematically, one would be justified in calling them tissue antigens. However, they are generally designated by the term "leucocyte antigens."

Family studies have been especially helpful in analyzing the HL-A locus. Such studies revealed that many antigens which had no apparent association in a random population were linked to markers known to be determined by the HL-A locus, and that the association of others was closer than believed initially. Much of the advantage of these family studies stemmed from the fact that the *haplotypes* * of the parents could be deduced from the antigenic patterns or "profiles" of their children (see Table 2.1).

Family studies also made it possible to determine the probability that given pairs of related individuals (parent-sib or sib-sib) will be HL-A compatible—a factor of considerable importance in the selection of donors for organ transplantation. Obviously, by serological means, it is frequently easy within families to match siblings so that they have identical haplotypes. It simply requires using certain antigenic markers to follow the inheritance of the particular chromosome that bears the HL-A locus.

Dr. Van Rood and his colleagues serologically classified the HL-A phenotypes of the members of forty families. They found that the frequency of the ten alleles most regularly encountered in the eighty parents ranged from 3 to 14%. In twenty-six of these forty families, the parents were heterozygous for *different* HL-A alleles. Thus, in such families, although there was a one-in-four chance that two children would receive the same allele from each parent and so be HL-A compatible, in no instance could any of the children be of the *same* HL-A genotype as either parent. In ten families the parents shared at least one allele, making it possible (the chance again being one in four) for identical parent-child HL-A compatible combinations to occur. The remaining four families comprised one parent who was homozygous at the HL-A locus and the other who was heterozygous (but for different alleles). Consequently,

---

* Dr. Ceppellini introduced the term "haplotype" for the antigens of one HL-A unit of genetic information (i.e., those associated with one chromosome) which corresponds to half the phenotype for a fully expressed co-dominant system.

Table 2.1

Illustrating the way in which family studies with typing sera provide evidence of the association of certain HL-A specificities. The father possesses antigens 1, 2, 4, 15, and 19. The mother lacks all of these except antigen 4. Consequently, the children can only have inherited the genetic determinants of antigens 1, 2, 15, and 19 from their father. Since the children have either antigens 1, 2, and 4 or 15 and 19, this indicates that all these antigens are determined by the same genetic locus. Furthermore, it follows that antigens 1, 2, and 4 are determined by one chromosomal region (A), and 15 and 19 by the same region on the homologous chromosome (B). By a similar line of reasoning, one can work out the antigens determined by equivalent chromosomal regions (C) and (D) in the mother. (Based on Batchelor, J.R. 1969. Brit. J. Hosp. Med. 2:(1199–1202.)

Father	A B	1, 2, 4 15, 19	
Mother	C D	4, 5 18	
Sib 1		15, 19 18	B D
Sib 2		15, 19 4, 5	B C
Sib 3		15, 19 4, 5	B C
Sib 4		1, 2, 4 4, 5	A C
Sib 5		1, 2, 4 4, 5	A C

although this situation precluded the possibility that any child could be of the same HL-A genotype as either parent, there was a one-in-two chance that two siblings would be of simlar HL-A types. The chances of identical parent-child and sib-sib HL-A genotypes arising from these different matings are summarized in Table 2.2.

Of course it should be appreciated that inasmuch as Van Rood's classification of HL-A genotypes was made on the basis of serotyping alone it is at best tentative; i.e., the use of additional typing sera could very well reveal previously uncovered differences. Thus parents categorized as homozygous might be shown in more complete studies to be heterozygous and parents who presently are believed to share one haplotype could have completely different haplotypes. On the other hand, siblings classified as HL-A identical on the basis of genetic and serological analyses are unlikely

Table 2.2

The relation between the HL-A genotypes of the parents and the expected frequency of occurrence of identical HL-A leucocyte groups in parent → child and sib → sib pairs in the family. The HL-A alleles of the parents are designated a, b, c, and d.

Genotypes of parents	*Genotypes of offspring*	*Donor-recipient combination*	*Grafts expected to be identical with host at HL-A locus (%)*
ab × cd	ac ad bc bd	parent → child	0
		sib → sib	25
ab × ad	aa ab ad bd	parent → child	25
		sib → sib	25
aa × bc	ab ac ab ac	parent → child	0
		sib → sib	50

to be reclassified—except, of course, for recombination which might have gone undetected in initial studies.

Despite the limitation of trying to match unrelated individuals with respect to their haplotypes by means of serotyping, the results of several recent studies have shown that there is a significant correlation between the degree of leucocyte matching that can be attained by currently available reagents and the survival of kidney transplants from unrelated cadaver donors in man.

In Vivo and In Vitro Histocompatibility Tests

So far we've only considered serological methods of histocompatibility testing and viewed them for the light they shed on the genetics of histocompatibility systems of man. There are, however, several in vivo or in vitro biological tests which have been devised for histocompatibility matching, some of which are now mainly of historic interest and others which are still useful in certain situations despite their inability to recognize specific antigens.

The ideal solution to the clinical homograft problem would be to devise a discriminatory typing procedure enabling donor and recipient to be matched so well that the latter is confronted by *no* foreign transplantation antigens. Unfortunately, such is the complexity of the genetic polymorphisms involved in human populations that, with the exception of identical twins, this ideal solution is virtually unattainable. Indeed, it is exceedingly difficult to match *unrelated* individuals with respect to their HL-A genotypes, apart from the multitude of other determinants of transplantation antigens. Nevertheless, the need to be able to select the most compatible donor for a given recipient (or the most compatible recipient in a "waiting" panel for an organ graft from a given cadaver donor) is of crucial importance if the results of organ homotransplantation are to be improved and their benefits made more widely available.

The best indication that some kind of genotyping procedure might be able to prolong the survival of renal and other homografts in man was the finding that grafts derived from parents or siblings survived on sibling hosts for significantly longer than grafts from unrelated donors. Intrafamilial grafts usually require lower dosages of immunosuppressive drugs and, consequently, many of the complications associated with the administration of these agents are avoided. Since a person inherits half his genetic material from his father and half from his mother, it follows that with parent-to-sibling grafts not more than 50% of the histocompatibility factors present in the graft can be foreign to the host (the actual percentage depends upon the number of histocompatibility loci at which the parent is heterozygous). On the other hand, the degree of possible genetic variation between siblings is much greater since each may have received selections of parental genetic material which are either very similar or very dissimilar to each other. Thus in large families, one would expect that some sib-sib combinations would be more compatible and other sib-sib combinations would be *less* compatible than parent-to-offspring combinations.

The simplest and most direct means conceivable for selecting the best kidney donor for a given recipient from an available panel is to remove an "indicator" skin graft from each possible donor and place it upon the recipient. The donor of the longest-lived graft would be the one of choice. The major objection to this procedure is that, short of finding an almost completely compatible donor, it unavoidably sensitizes the recipient to his future donor's antigens, exacerbating the problem of immunosuppression.

To eliminate the undesirable hazards of sensitizing the recipient, two variant skin-test grafting procedures have been devised and employed on a small scale.

The Inverse Skin Grafting Method involves the transplantation of skin grafts *from* the propositus to each member of the donor panel. The donor chosen is the one upon whom the propositus' skin survives longest on the basis of the assumption that this graft shares more antigens in common with the propositus than do the other grafts.

The Third-Man Test (illustrated in Fig. 2.1) was developed independently by Drs. Wilson, Henry, and Merrill in Boston and by Dr. Mathé and his associates in Paris. It entails, first, challenging an "indifferent" host,

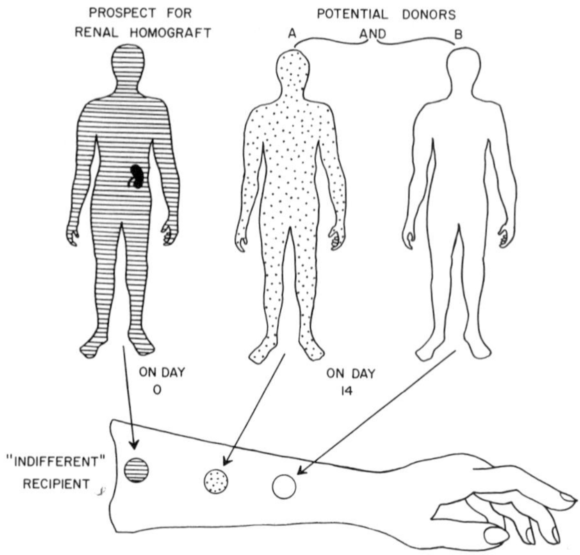

Fig. 2.1. The third-man test. A normal "indifferent" individual is first given a skin homograft from the person needing a renal homograft. Fourteen days later, when this graft has been rejected, the indifferent host is given a skin homograft from each of the possible renal homograft donors, A and B. If A's graft is rejected more rapidly than that from B, this is an indication that the patient and A share important transplantation antigens.

H, with a skin graft from the propositus, R, and allowing it to be rejected. Following this, H is challenged with skin grafts from the panel of possible donors, D_1, D_2, D_3, etc. The individual in the donor series whose graft is rejected the most rapidly is selected as the kidney donor on the premise that the prompt rejection of his test graft is indicative of the sharing of at least one important antigen with the recipient.

Unfortunately, despite their common advantage of not sensitizing the propositus, both of these tests share the serious shortcomings that they are able to select only individuals who *share* histocompatibility antigens, rather than individuals who *differ* with respect to important antigens. Thus, in the inverse grafting method, if the propositus was homozygous at a major histocompatibility locus, A, being of genotype AA, and one of the donor panel was AA′, the latter might well be selected as the optimal donor. In this case, however, his kidney would confront the recipient with a major alien transplantation antigen. Likewise, in the third-man test, if the kidney recipient is homozygous, AA, at a major histocompatibility locus, and the "indifferent" host happens to be A′A′, skin from a donor who is heterozygous at this locus, i.e., is AA′, would undergo accelerated rejection and yet be markedly incompatible with the AA propositus.

In 1963 Brent and Medawar presented highly encouraging results from a method of histocompatibility matching which they'd developed and tested in an outbred population of guinea pigs. In this procedure, illustrated in Fig. 2.2, known as the Normal Lymphocyte Transfer (NLT) Test, small aliquots of a viable suspension of lymphocytes prepared from the blood of an intended graft recipient (R) are injected intradermally

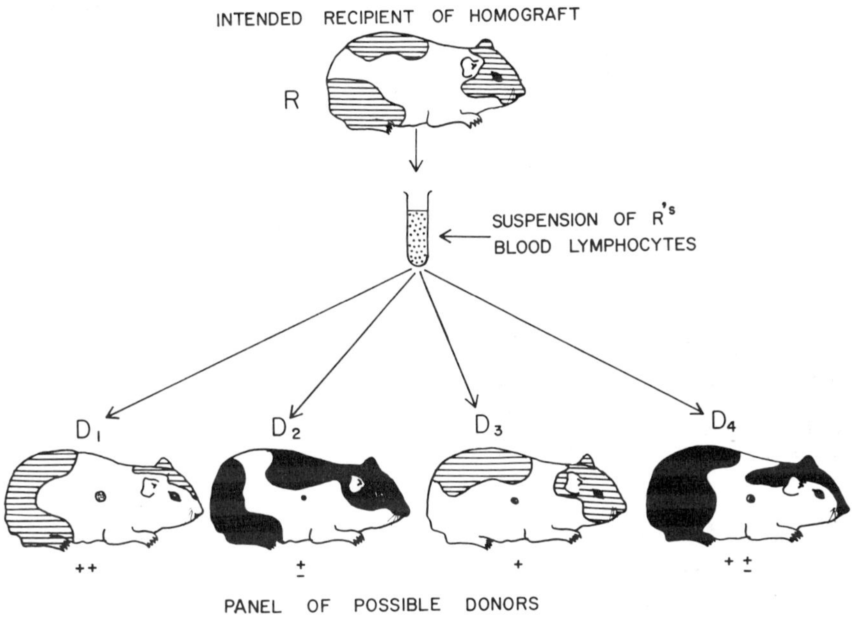

Fig. 2.2. Illustrating the principle of the Normal Lymphocyte Transfer typing test for selecting the most compatible skin homograft donor from an available panel. Of the four possible donors, the one which displays the minimal cutaneous reactivity when injected intradermally with the intended recipient's lymphocytes, D_2, with the score ±, would be the donor of choice. D_1, which gave a reaction of intensity score ++, would be the donor presenting the strongest histoincompatibility.

into the members of a possible donor panel, D_1, D_2, D_3, etc. Small, erythematous wheals develop at the inoculation sites after a delay of eight to twenty-four hours, reaching their peak intensities after about forty-eight hours. Various lines of evidence attested to the fact that these tuberculin-like reactions reflect graft-versus-host reactivities (see Chapter 11) on the part of R's immunologically competent lymphocytes against the foreign transplantation antigens confronting them in the skins of the donor panel, D_1, D_2, D_3, etc. It therefore followed that their magnitudes should give some indication of the intensity of the reactions to be expected if R is challenged with skin grafts from D_1, D_2, D_3, etc. Confirmatory evidence for this thesis was afforded by the finding that there was indeed a close correlation between the magnitudes of the reactions incited by the lymphocytes from R in the skins of these various animals and the order of rejection of skin grafts from them subsequently transplanted to R. Thus, if the strongest skin reactions were incited by R's cells inoculated into D_2, skin from D_2 to R had a shorter survival time than did skin from other members of the donor panel.

These interesting findings furnished unequivocal evidence that the problem of histocompatibility matching was, in principle, soluble. Furthermore, since men, like guinea pigs, exhibit good cutaneous hypersensitivity reactions to appropriate antigens, it seemed likely that the NLT test would also prove applicable in this species.

Unfortunately, despite the fact that good skin reactions attend the performance of NLT tests in man, their prognostic value has been rather disappointing. In Gray's and Russell's experience, although the test could reliably eliminate grossly incompatible donors, it was unable to select, consistently, the best donor from a panel of blood relatives. It is also interesting to note that the transfer of lymphocytes across an ABO blood group barrier appears to have no significant effect on the size of the reaction although, as already stated, this barrier does exert an adverse influence on the survival of homografts.

A number of different factors contribute to the disappointing results obtained with the NLT test in man. From the viewpoint of its capacity to select kidney donors, a serious complication is the fact that lymphocytes from uremic patients may display impaired reactivity, which is probably not due to the uremia per se, but to the intoxicated and debilitated state of the patient. For this reason, lymphocytes from uremic individuals tend to indicate a higher percentage of good donors than is actually the case. The size of the NLT reactions is also dependent upon the general condition of the potential organ donors. Thus patients with certain kinds of malignancies, including Hodgkin's disease, develop smaller reactions on receipt of lymphocytes from healthy donors than do healthy recipients. Despite its poor discriminatory power in man and the risk of inadvertently transmitting infections along with the lymphocyte inocula, the NLT test is certainly better than no test at all. For this reason, it should not be entirely dismissed as a matching procedure.

The Irradiated Hamster Test devised by Ramseier and Streilein (see Fig. 2.3) is somewhat similar to the NLT test in concept, though it has the decided advantage of not requiring the exposure of a panel of potential organ donors to cells from the propositus. This assay takes advantage of the facts that (1) Syrian hamsters, like guinea pigs and man, are capable of expressing homograft sensitivity in the form of local cutaneous hypersensitivity reactions of the delayed type and (2) the integument of lethally

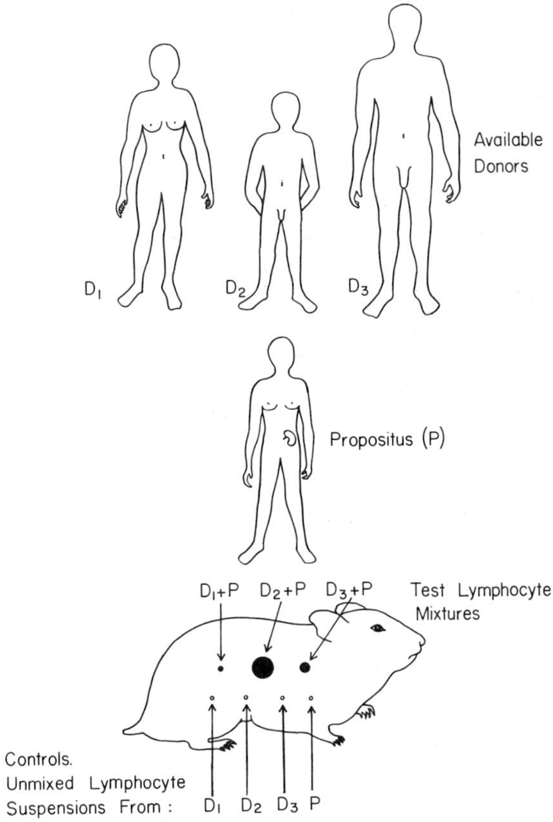

Fig. 2.3. Illustrating the principle of the irradiated hamster test.

X-irradiated albino hamsters, which are themselves incapable of any reactivity against foreign cells, furnishes a favorable sustaining milieu for the study of homograft hypersensitivity at the cellular level when the essential cellular components are added. Consequently, when a suspension of viable hamster lymph node cells is mixed with a suspension of homologous cells and injected into the skin of an irradiated hamster, a delayed cutaneous response develops at the site. The intensity of this reaction can be shown, by skin grafting tests, to be dependent upon the degree of antigenic disparity between the immunologically competent cells and their homologous target cells. What is even more remarkable is that the skin of these irradiated hamsters also provides an effective milieu for the expression of homograft reactivities in which the cellular reactants are derived from members of an *alien* or heterologous donor species. Thus mixtures of human lymphocytes obtained by fractionation of the blood of two unrelated donors, when inoculated intracutaneously into irradiated hamsters, react in a manner closely resembling that of mixtures of hamster cells.

The results of this test system, which has been thoroughly investigated for skin graft matching in rats and mice, and to a lesser extent in humans, are similar to those obtained with the NLT test. They indicate that, while the test may be useful in ruling out grossly incompatible donors, it is not very discriminatory where lesser degrees of histoincompatibility are involved. Moreover, as described, the test is a two-way test, indicating not only the reactivity of the propositus' cells against those of the potential donor, but also that of the latter's cells against the alien antigens of the propositus. Although it is claimed that the latter reactivity can be abolished by the simple expedient of incubating the cells of the potential donor in Tyrode's solution for two hours at 37°C, further efforts are necessary to evaluate the influence of this on the reliability of the test.

Undoubtedly the greatest weakness of both the NLT and irradiated hamster test is the dearth of information concerning their ability to match individuals with respect to alleles at the HL-A locus. Indeed, it is primarily because of this shortcoming that these procedures are, at least for the present, subordinate to the final biological matching procedure we shall now consider—the so-called *Mixed Leucocyte Culture (MLC) Test.*

The Mixed Leucocyte Culture Test, developed by Bain and Lowenstein and by Hirschorn and Bach, like the NLT test and the irradiated hamster test, also turns upon the immunological competence of blood lymphocytes. It is based upon the fact that, when these cells are exposed, in vitro, to HL-A incompatible cellular isoantigens (usually viable leucocytes, for convenience), some of them transform into large basophilic, blast-like cells which take up tritiated thymidine and divide. On the other hand, when both co-donors of such mixed cell suspensions have the same HL-A alleles, no significant reactivity can be measured in terms of the uptake and incorporation of tritiated thymidine. Although, as described, the test is two-directional—A's lymphocytes reacting against B's and vice versa—it can easily be made undirectional. Incubation of the potential organ donor's lymphocytes with Mitomycin C, prior to admixture with the recipient's cells, inhibits mitotic activity on the part of the former.

The MLC test affords a very reliable means of selecting HL-A compatible donors for given recipients. It can also be used in family studies to identify individuals who differ only with regard to one of their HL-A haplotypes since, when certain dosages of cells are placed in mixed cultures together, the cells of siblings differing from the responding sib by *both* alleles at the HL-A locus stimulate a greater in vitro response than do cells from sibs differing by only one allele at this locus. Although the clinical significance of this observation remains to be evaluated, recent data do indicate that the survival times of skin grafts in combinations differing for two HL-A alleles are shorter than in cases differing for one allele.*

This test has been subjected to critical evaluation in mice and rats, where the availability of isogenic strains and their F_1 and R_2 progeny have made it possible to study cell mixtures which preclude the undesirable two-way reactions. One of these studies, illustrated in Fig. 2.4, is particularly pertinent since it indicates the close similarity of the results obtainable in rats and in man. (DA × Lewis) F_1 hybrids rats, which are $Ag\text{-}B^4/Ag\text{-}B^1$,

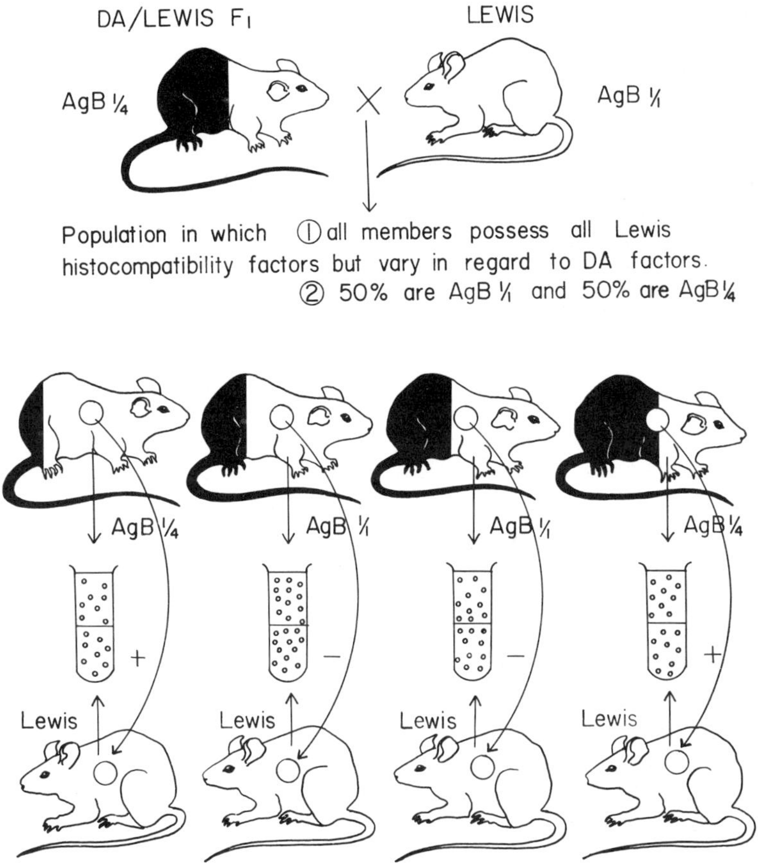

Fig. 2.4. Illustrating the experimental procedure which established that, in the rat: (1) in vitro Mixed Leucocyte Reactivity occurs only where histoincompatibility at the Ag-B locus prevails and (2) this in vitro reactivity does not necessarily provide a measure of the intensity of skin homograft reactivity.

---

* This concept of a "one-allele different" donor is, of course, meaningful only within a family, since it is possible that a two-allele different unrelated donor could be a better donor than a one-allele different related donor.

were backcrossed to Lewis ($Ag\text{-}B^1/Ag\text{-}B^1$) animals to produce an R_2 backcross population. All members of this population have one complete set of Lewis chromosomes and are therefore genetically tolerant of Lewis histocompatibility antigens. Furthermore, this population comprises equal numbers of homozygous $Ag\text{-}B^1/Ag\text{-}B^1$ and heterozygous $Ag\text{-}B^1/Ag\text{-}B^4$ animals which possess different complements of other specific DA histocompatibility genes. When leucocytes from these R_2 animals were placed in mixed culture with Lewis leucocytes, it was found that incorporation of tritiated thymidine occurred *only* when the R_2 co-donor was $Ag\text{-}B^1/Ag\text{-}B^4$. That is, $Ag\text{-}B^1/Ag\text{-}B^1$ Lewis leucocytes responded to only those R_2 cells that confronted them with an $Ag\text{-}B^4$ isoantigen, regardless of the other histocompatibility antigens present and in spite of the fact that some Lewis rats rejected skin homografts from $Ag\text{-}B^1/Ag\text{-}B^1$ R_2 donors as promptly as they rejected grafts from $Ag\text{-}B^1/Ag\text{-}B^4$ R_2 donors. Nevertheless, compatibility at the Ag-B locus proved to be important in that it facilitated the prolongation of skin homograft survival by immunosuppressive therapy.

Since in man all the available evidence is consistent with the premise that the MLC test is HL-A specific, its utilization in family and population studies has yielded some interesting information. For example, family studies employing this test, in conjunction with serological leucocyte typing procedures, have revealed that most of the antigens measured by currently available leukocyte antisera are part of the HL-A system. Serological data and MLC tests have also revealed that the HL-A system is highly polymorphic. For example, when twenty-two unrelated individuals were intensively studied at a Histocompatibility Workshop held in Italy in 1967, it was found that all forty-four HL-A alleles of these individuals had *different* combinations of antigens associated with them. Indeed, this polymorphism of the HL-A locus constitutes one of the most serious obstacles in the way of finding HL-A compatible organs, especially when these are to be obtained from cadavers. While cooperation between surgical units should enhance the likelihood that an available organ will reach a compatible host, the potential value of cadaver transplants will probably not be realized until means of preserving organs for at least some days, and preferably for weeks or months, have been developed. Then, and only then, will it be possible to ensure that every suitable cadaver organ which becomes available for transplantation is used to the best advantage by being sent to a center in which there happens to be a highly compatible recipient.*

---

* On the basis of their recent computer analysis of the frequency of thirteen HL-A specificities in 180 unrelated individuals, Dr. Festenstein and his associates in London concluded that, with a single kidney donor and a panel of only twelve unrelated putative recipients, an identical match is very unlikely to occur. With a pool size of 120 recipients, one would expect

Some idea of the importance of HL-A compatibility so far as the prognosis of renal homotransplantation is concerned can be gained from a report by Rapaport and his associates. They found that 56% of patients reeciving HL-A incompatible kidney grafts from living blood relatives had either rejected their grafts or were ranked as being in poor clinical condition after 12 months. The comparable figure for HL-A compatible grafts was 16%. These figures were based on a total of 50 patients. At 28 months post-operation, the difference in a group of 37 patients was even more striking: 69% of the HL-A incompatible kidneys had either been rejected or were at a late stage of rejection. But only 8% of the compatible grafts were in this category; the remaining 92% continuing to survive. Essentially similar findings have been reported for organ grafts from unrelated living or cadaver donors.

Although the various matching procedures described above have facilitated the selection of compatible donors for individuals requiring organ or tissue transplants, their usefulness is limited by a number of factors. First, their application is almost completely restricted to situations where family members are available as donors, since only in such instances are individuals readily available who are compatible with the propositi with regard to their HL-A antigens. Second, their application is limited when the problem is to find suitable recipients for cadaver organs, or to matching donors and recipients who do not live in close proximity. Finally, and probably most important, they are procedures which are specific for the particular combination of individuals for which they are employed, i.e., a reaction of A's cells with B's or C's cells will reveal little, if anything, about B's reaction to C's cells or C's reaction to B's cells. For these reasons there can be no doubt that ultimately the most effective and probably the only worthwhile procedure for donor selection will be serologically based leucocyte typing. Indeed, the day may not be too far off when individuals can be typed for their important histocompatibility antigens as easily and routinely as they are presently typed for their blood group factors so that, at death, their organs may be readily available for suitable, predetermined recipients. However, until this time arrives, the information obtainable from the MLC test and from some of the other matching procedures described in this chapter will probably continue to be helpful, alongside the

---

to find at least two who were mismatches for fewer than two antigens for a single donor. Using this criterion, it should be possible to use every available kidney. To ensure having one identical match for a given donor kidney, a pool of upwards of 240 potential hosts would be required—a figure close to the total number of patients being maintained on chronic hemodialysis in the greater London area.

results of leukocyte typing, in selecting the most compatible donor for a given recipient.*

REFERENCES

Bach, F. H. 1970. Transplantation: pairing of donor and recipient. Science 168:1170–1179.

Bach, F. H. 1969. Histocompatibility in man. Genetic and practical considerations, p. 201–240. *In* Progress in human genetics, VI. Grune and Stratton, New York.

Dausset, J., and F. T. Rapaport. 1968. Blood group determinants of human histocompatibility, p. 383–393. *In* F. T. Rapaport and J. Dausset [ed.] Human transplantation. Grune and Stratton, New York and London.

Histocompatibility testing. 1965. Munksgaard, Copenhagen.

Histocompatibility testing. 1967. Munksgaard, Copenhagen.

Nelson, S. D., and P. S. Russell. 1968. In vivo histocompatibility testing, p. 394–405. *In* F. T. Rapaport and J. Dausset [ed.] Human transplantation. Grune and Stratton, New York and London.

* A recent analysis by Van Rood and Eijsvoogel is particularly revealing in presenting some idea of the reliability of current serological typing procedures in evaluating HL-A compatibility. These investigators screened the HL-A typing records of 500 *unrelated* individuals with a computer and selected four individuals who had been typed identically for HL-A antigens. Two-way and one-way mixed lymphocyte culture tests between all possible combinations of these four individuals were then carried out. Of these four individuals, one HL-A identical pair was confirmed by the MLC test.

Chapter 3

Weak Histocompatibility Factors

So far we have confined ourselves almost entirely to a consideration of the so-called major histoincompatibilities of mice, rats, and man. Although these incompatibilities are of special interest because of the predominant role they play in all manifestations of transplantation immunity, they nevertheless represent only a minority of the total number of histocompatibility factors present in most species. Knowledge of both the genetic determination and the immunological properties of "weak" transplantation antigens has increased considerably during the past decade, partly as a consequence of the increasing availability of appropriate experimental subjects in different species, and partly because of increasing interest in them for the following reasons:

1. It has become obvious that some of the general tenets of transplantation immunology, as formulated from studies on "strong" histocompatibility differences, do not apply where only weak histoincompatibilities are involved.
2. As histocompatibility typing improves, hopefully, clinicians will be mainly concerned with the abrogation of weak rather than strong histoincompatibility reactions.
3. It is relatively simple to induce tolerance of homografts in situations where nonmajor locus differences prevail.

One important principle which has emerged is that "minor" histocompatibility loci cannot be ranked or categorized in terms of the potency of their antigenic products, since this is a function of the particular interallelic combination involved. For example, the MST's of skin grafts exchanged between mice which differ only with respect to their H-1 genotype may differ by more than two hundred days, depending upon which strain serves as the donor and which the recipient. Moreover, with some of these combinations allelic *dosage* effects are demonstrable, i.e., grafts which are heterozygous for the foreign allele may survive longer than grafts which are homozygous for it.

Where only minor histoincompatibilities exist it has been found that the later the time of onset of skin graft rejection, the longer it usually takes for the process to be completed. For example, Hildemann and Walford at U.C.L.A., working with a population of outbred Syrian hamsters made this observation: Whereas acute rejection of skin homografts was usually complete within 2½ days of its overt onset, chronic rejections, where signs of incompatibility did not appear until the grafts had been in place for about one hundred days, usually required several months for their completion. This finding sustains the important empirical principle that the longer a homograft remains fully viable, the greater the probability that it will continue to survive. In other words, if two individuals both have healthy skin homografts of fifteen days' and of fifty days' standing, respectively, the probability of the second graft surviving an additional twenty-five days (say) is much greater than that of the first graft surviving for the *same* amount of additional time.

Furthermore, the weaker the immunogenetic disparity between donor and host strain combinations, the greater the variation in survival times of individual skin grafts. For example, with one congenic resistant strain combination in which the MST of skin grafts was about 15 days, individual survival scores ranged from 11 to 23 days, whereas in another combination with an MST of 38 days, individual scores fell within the range of 24 to 153 days.

Where *strong* histoincompatibilities are involved, there is a weak but definite *inverse* relationship between graft size or "dosage" and its expectation of survival—small grafts tending to live longer than large grafts. Indeed, as already mentioned (see page 13), this dosage effect was one of the crucial pieces of evidence Medawar cited in favor of the thesis that homograft rejection is an immunological phenomenon. However, where only *weak* histoincompatibilities are involved, small grafts may be rejected eventually whereas larger grafts may survive indefinitely under similar experimental conditions. This dosage effect, which becomes more conspicuous the weaker the degree of donor-recipient incompatibility, is well illustrated by findings of Lapp and Bliss of McGill University. They compared the survival times of H-1 locus incompatible skin grafts of four different size ranges or "dosages"—6 to 12 mg, 13 to 50 mg, 51 to 125 mg, and 126 to 300 mg. These investigators found that: (1) the *larger* the grafts the longer the MST's; (2) there was an allelic dosage effect—larger grafts lived even longer if they were derived from heterozygous instead of homozygous donors; and (3) this allelic dosage effect persisted even when heterozygous and homozygous skin grafts were placed on the *same* hosts at the same time. It follows from the last observation that, regardless of the mechanism responsible for prolonging the survival of the larger grafts, grafts from heterozygous donors are less vulnerable to attack than those from homozygous donors.

Lappé and his associates have recently shown that a similar situation also occurs when mice are grafted simultaneously with *both* large and small skin grafts from the same donor, i.e., the large grafts persist significantly longer than the contralaterally placed small grafts. This suggests that an immune response of a given magnitude takes significantly longer to destroy a large graft than a small one and that, in some instances, a slow chronic rejection might permit the occurrence of a significant amount of cellular repair and replacement leading to the appearance of "permanent survival" in the absence of "true tolerance."

The principle that where only weak histoincompatibilities prevail small grafts may be rejected whereas larger grafts may persist must be taken into consideration in evaluating the results of tests, such as the F_2 test, designed to estimate the number of histocompatibility loci for a given species (see Chapter 1). Bailey and Mobraaten have reported that BALB/c and C57BL/6 mice differ by as many as twenty-nine to thirty-two histocompatibility genes—an estimate greatly in excess of the fifteen to seventeen histocompatibility loci for mice arrived at by other investigators. This high figure almost certainly resulted from the employment of exceedingly small tail skin grafts. Had skin grafts of conventional size been employed, many of them may have escaped rejection when only weak incompatibilities prevailed. Thus Bailey and Mobraaten's estimate is probably more accurate than those obtained by more conventional grafting procedures.

There is a considerable body of evidence that, in general, females give more vigorous immunological responses than males. This has proved to be the case with homograft reactions too, especially where weak transplantation antigens are involved. However, this sex difference is not always evident nor does it appear to be correlated with the strength of the histocompatibility barrier. For example, the MST of skin grafts transplanted from $H\text{-}3^a$ mice to $H\text{-}3^b$ animals may be twenty-one or thirty days, depending upon whether the hosts are females or males, respectively. However, in another CR combination, $H\text{-}4^a \longrightarrow H\text{-}4^b$, grafts have an MST of about one hundred and twenty days regardless of the sex of the host. The greatest influence of sex on the MST of skin grafts occurs with the CR combination $H\text{-}10^b \longrightarrow H\text{-}10^a$. Here the MST of grafts to female recipients is seventy-one days while that of grafts to males exceeds three hundred days.

One of the most important facts about weak transplantation antigens is that they can act *synergistically*—the MST of skin grafts confronting their hosts with two alien histocompatibility factors may be significantly shorter than when graft and host differ by only one or the other of the factors on its own. However, this cumulative effect prevails only when the disparity between the strengths of the constituent antigens is not too great. It is lost when the ratio between their MST's is greater than 3:1. A good example of this phenomenon is provided by the fate of skin grafts differing from their hosts at the H-4 and H-11 loci in mice. The MST of $H\text{-}4^a$ skin grafts on congenic $H\text{-}4^b$ animals is 120 days, and that of $H\text{-}11^b$ grafts on $H\text{-}11^a$ hosts is 164 days. However, when donor and host differ with respect to *both* of these weak factors, i.e., in the combination $H\text{-}4^a$, $H\text{-}11^b \longrightarrow H\text{-}4^b$, $H\text{-}11^a$, the MST is reduced to 58 days. On the other hand, there is no cumulative effect in the reverse direction, $H\text{-}4^b$, $H\text{-}11^a \longrightarrow H\text{-}4^a$, $H\text{-}11^b$, inasmuch as the MST of $H\text{-}4^b$ skin on $H\text{-}4^a$ mice is 25 days and that from $H\text{-}11^a$ donors to $H\text{-}11^b$ hosts is 78 days.

Cumulative effects are also demonstrable in rats. For example, Lewis strain animals reject skin grafts from Fischer donors just as promptly as they reject grafts from BN donors, in spite of the fact that Lewis and Fischer animals are Ag-B compatible, while Lewis and BN rats are not.

These additive effects may be important clinically insofar as they can enable individually weak and ineffective immunogens to become important through their combined influence. Of course there is a limit to this principle in the sense that, once a graft has a sufficient isoantigenic constitution to evoke a maximal immunologic response from a host, the addition of further immunogens to the graft would not curtail its survival any further.

The capacity of histocompatibility antigens to act synergistically may also explain the apparent strength of the H-2 locus and its homologues in rats and man. Since these loci seem to comprise a series of pseudoalleles, each of which probably determines a single antigenic specificity, their potency could result from the concerted action of all these factors, some of which, individually, are of medium or even weak immunogenicity. Indeed, Dr. J. Klein of the Czechoslovakian Academy of Sciences has obtained some experimental support for this interpretation. Utilizing the appropriate congenic-resistant line combinations, as well as their F_1 hybrids, he found that skin grafts which confronted their murine hosts with only a single foreign H-2 antigenic specificity survived longer than when two or more differences at this locus prevailed.

The basis for these synergistic effects is still unknown. It is possible that when a strong and a weak antigen occur on the *same* cellular vehicle, the host's response against the strong antigen, which culminates in the destruction of the cell, interferes with or preempts its potential response against the weak immunogen. However, when two or more immunogens of approximately equivalent potency are present on the same cell, immunity may develop against them all *concurrently* and thus lead to more rapid destruction of the target cell.

The H-Y Locus

There is one weak antigen that deserves special consideration, not only because it represents an exception to the rule that grafts exchanged between members of an isogenic population are always accepted, but also because of its special usefulness for a variety of purposes.

In 1955 Eichwald and Silmser discovered that in certain inbred strains of mice, isografts from males to females were rejected, whereas grafts from males to males, or females to males were always accepted. Subsequently it was shown that this sex-associated incompatibility also applies in rats. Since the only genetic difference between male and female members of an inbred strain is that males have the Y chromosome, of which there is no homologue in females, the simplest explanation for this incompatibility is that there is a histocompatibility antigen(s) determined by a locus on the Y chromosome.* Alternatively, it could be argued that, although the so-called Y factor occurs only in males, its synthesis is *autosomally* determined, i.e., the genetic determinant is present in both males and females but is only able to express itself in the presence of a Y chromosome or, more specifically, in the presence of male hormones (or in the absence of female hormones). However, no evidence for this latter contention has been forthcoming and several findings tell against it. For example, skin grafts from neonatal C57BL/6 female donors transplanted orthotopically to adult C57BL/6 male hosts and maintained there for at least 100 days—a period which should afford ample opportunity for them to produce the Y antigen, if hormonal factors alone are involved in its synthesis—do not express the antigen. This is evidenced by the observation that, if such long-standing neonatal female grafts on male hosts are excised and transferred to either normal isogenic females or to specifically presensitized females (animals which had previously received and rejected two successive male skin isografts), they are permanently accepted.

Celada and Welshons have also carried out experiments, the results of which are not only consistent with Y linkage, but also rule out the possibilities that the Y antigen results from the presence of only one X chromosome, or that its production is suppressed by two X chromosomes. These investigators used an exceptional stock of mice in which some females possessed only a single X chromosome (XO) and a single exceptional male mouse which had two X chromosomes and one Y chromosome (XXY). Since these mice were not isogenic, the role of the Y chromosome could

* An analogous situation occurs in chickens except that, inasmuch as in birds it is the female sex which is heterogametic, males react against female isografts.

not be tested directly by challenging females with male skin grafts. Instead, the presence or absence of the Y factor was demonstrated indirectly by the capacity of tissues bearing it to immunize. Normal females were inoculated with spleen cells of XO or XXY origin and subsequently challenged with isogenic male spleen cells from donors presensitized to rat erythrocytes. The demonstrably impaired production of anti-erythrocyte antibody by these transferred cells—a reflection of their accelerated destruction—was taken as evidence of presensitization of the hosts to the Y antigen. While cells from XXY males immunized normal females with regard to isologous male spleen cells, cells from XO females did not. It is therefore evident that the Y factor results from the presence of a Y chromosome and not from the absence of a second X chromosome.

In the light of the findings just described, it seems likely that although the synthesis of the Y antigen is determined by a Y-linked histocompatibility locus (or loci) hormonal factors may influence its immunogenicity. Evidence for this interpretation is provided by the observation that castrating males at birth or shortly thereafter or raising neonatal male skin on adult females significantly reduces the antigenicity of the skin as attested by its extended survival when transferred to adult females.

In both mice and rats the ability of females to reject isografts of male skin varies from strain to strain. In mice, for example, virtually 100% of C57BL/6 females and about 75% of strain A females reject male skin isografts, with MST's of about twenty-five and fifty days, respectively. By contrast, CBA and AU strain females usually accept such grafts. The occurrence of this interstrain diversity of the faculty to respond to this antigen is surprising since the specificity of the Y factor is the same in male mice of *all* stocks so far tested. The last statement rests upon the following observations:

1. Skin grafts are accepted when exchanged between reciprocal F_1 hybrid males, i.e., males which are identical in every respect except for the origin of their X and Y chromosomes. For example, the F_1 hybrid male offspring derived from mating C57BL/6 males with CBA females receive their X chromosome from their CBA mothers and their Y chromosome from their C57BL/6 fathers. On the other hand, F_1 males born from C57BL/6 mothers and CBA fathers have a C57BL/6 X chromosome and a CBA Y chromosome. Consequently one would expect that, if different alleles occurred at the H-Y locus, skin grafts exchanged between such reciprocally produced males would not always be accepted. This is not the case except, of course, when the strains employed have *different* X-linked histocompatibility alleles.*

* Following the discovery of the male specific antigen in the mouse, attempts were made to determine whether there was an X-linked locus in

2. Evidence for the identity of the Y antigen in male mice of *all* strains is afforded by the fact that adult females are sensitized against male skin isografts following exposure to male tissue derived from completely unrelated *male* mice. Indeed, this was apparent from the work of Celada and Welshons who found that females inoculated with homologous male spleen cells manifested an immune response when challenged with isologous male spleen cells.

3. What is probably the most conclusive evidence as to the constancy of the Y antigen in different strains had been provided by studies on the induction of tolerance (see Chapter 10). If neonatal C57BL/6 females are inoculated with suspensions of living bone marrow cells from C3H, CBA, AU, or A strain *males,* they are incapable of reacting against C57BL/6 male skin grafts transplanted to them in adult life. But if females are inoculated at birth with marrow cells from *female* donors of these various strains, they react normally against such grafts.

Attempts have been made, using the experimental designs outlined in items 2 and 3 above, to determine whether Y factors of mice and rats are antigenically similar. Adult C57BL/6 female mice were injected with spleen cells from adult male rats in the hope of eliciting sensitization against subsequent male skin isografts, but without success. Likewise, attempts to induce tolerance of male skin isografts in C57BL/6 females by injecting them at birth with male rat cells proved unsuccessful. Thus, so far, there is no convincing evidence of any cross-reactivity between the antigenic specificities determined by the Y chromosome in these two species.

In the absence of the existence of alleles at the H-Y locus, an explanation is required for the considerable interstrain differences in *penetrance* (as reflected by the percentage of male isografts which are rejected by females of a given strain) and *expressivity* (as indicated by the MST's of these rejected grafts). The most plausible premise is that the genotype of the female recipient determines her capacity to react against the male

---

this species. Initially these efforts were unsuccessful, but in retrospect this can probably be attributed to the fact that either the strains selected for these studies by chance carried identical X-linked factors, or the test skin grafts employed were too large. Thus Bailey finally did demonstrate that small tail skin grafts exchanged between reciprocally produced (C57BL $\times$ BALB/c)F_1 hybrid males were often rejected. Inasmuch as such grafts differ only with regard to the origin of their X and Y chromosomes, and subsequent experiments by Bailey ruled out any Y-chromosome influence, it is apparent that there are transplantation antigens determined by the X chromosome. These antigens are comparatively very weak and probably would have gone undetected had Bailey not employed very small tail skin grafts in his analysis; i.e., skin grafts of "normal" size are usually, if not always, accepted across such a barrier.

antigen. The existence of differences in the immunological response faculty of mice of different strains is well established, and there is a correlation between the response faculty of several strains and the tendency of their females to reject male skin isografts. Furthermore, some direct evidence for this premise has been obtained. Klein and Linder produced F_1 hybrids by mating CBA female mice (which only very rarely reject male skin isografts) with C57BL/6 males (a strain in which the penetrance of the Y factor is virtually 100%). All the F_1 females derived from this mating rejected grafts from CBA males, indicating that ability to react was introduced into the F_1 from the C57 strain. Male F_1 hybrids were then backcrossed to CBA females to produce a population of mice which varied with respect to the proportion of C57 and CBA genes they possessed although, of course, all had a full complement of CBA chromosomes. The proportion of backcross females able to reject grafts of CBA male skin was then determined as a means of estimating the number of independently segregating factors, derived from the C57 genome, which controlled reactivity against the male antigen. Eighty-five of 110 backcross females rejected grafts from male CBA donors. This 77% rejection ratio, in conjunction with the frequency of distribution of graft survival times, indicated that two autosomal dominant genes, each of which behaved independently, were in some way responsible for determining a female's ability to respond to the Y factor. However, since interpretation of multiple-factor situations is difficult, the actual number of factors involved should probably be regarded as tentative at present. Nevertheless, these interesting findings certainly suggest that the disparity in reactivity to the Y factor displayed by females of different strains is due to autosomally inherited modifying factors, factors that probably affect the machinery of immunological response. They also indicate that an animal's capacity to react to any immunogen may be influenced by polygenic factors unrelated to the determinants of transplantation antigens.

Another way in which the genetic background could influence the intensity of homograft reactions is by affecting the expression of antigens. This could be mediated by an ability of non-H (histocompatibility) genes to alter the amount of cellular antigen produced, its availability to the host's immune system, or the vulnerability of the graft to immune attack. Evidence for such an influence has recently been obtained from experiments concerned with the expression of the Y factor. This work was based on the premise that, since the specificity of the Y antigen is the *same* in male mice of all strains, F_1 hybrid females should reject male skin grafts from their parental strains or from F_1 hybrids with equal promptitude, unless the different genetic backgrounds of these donors can influence the expression of this antigen. Accordingly, different panels of C57BL/CBA F_1 hybrid females were challenged, respectively, with skin grafts from

C57BL and CBA male donors and from F_1 hybrid male donors whose Y chromosomes were derived from either the CBA or C57BL strains. In addition, male-to-female isografts were carried out on panels of CBA and C57BL animals and grafts were exchanged between reciprocal hybrid males to confirm the identity of the male antigen in the strains concerned. The results, summarized in Table 3.1, are interesting because they demon-

Table 3.1

Survival times of C57BL and CBA male skin grafts on C57BL and CBA female mice, respectively, and on C57/CBA F_1 hybrid females. All male skin isografts are rejected by C57BL females and are usually accepted by CBA females. However, F_1 hybrid females reject CBA male skin grafts and F_1 hybrid male skin grafts bearing a C57 or CBA Y chromosome much more frequently than they reject C57BL male skin grafts. This is attributed to the fact that, although the specificity of the Y antigen is the same in C57BL and CBA males, as evidenced by the acceptance of skin grafts exchanged between reciprocal F_1 hybrid males, its immunogenicity is stronger in the latter strain.

Donor male	*Recipient female*	*Number of recipients grafted*	*Distribution of graft survival times (days)* 15–24	25–50	51–75	76–100	>100	*Median survival time (days)*
C57	C57	21	11	9	1			25.6 ± 4.0
CBA	CBA	15			1	1	13	
C57	F_1	28	2	9	2	1	14	
CBA	F_1	30	18	11			1	24.2 ± 4.2
F_1(C57Y)	F_1	19	12	5	1	1		24.0 ± 5.5
F_1(CBAY)	F_1	18	11	5	1		1	23.0 ± 3.3
F_1(CBAY)	F_1(C57Y)	15					15	
F_1(C57Y)	F_1(CBAY)	14					14	

strate that, although the penetrance and expressivity of the Y factor are much more pronounced in C57BL mice than in CBA mice, the survival of C57BL male grafts on F_1 hybrid females was significantly longer (50% survived for more than one hundred days) than that of CBA male grafts on similar hosts (the majority of which are rejected within fifty days). Grafts from F_1 hybrid males were rejected as promptly as CBA male grafts, regardless of the origin of the Y chromosome, and, as anticipated, reciprocal male-to-male F_1 grafts survived indefinitely.

It is therefore evident that a donor's genetic background can influence the capacity of its tissue's Y antigen to elicit rejection when grafted. Furthermore, F_1 hybrid females rejected C57BL male skin grafts *less* rapidly than they rejected grafts from CBA males. This indicates that the more pronounced penetrance of the Y factor in C57BL mice must be due to the ability of C57BL females to develop a stronger response to male isografts than do CBA females.

The basis for the discrepancy in expression of the Y factor in these two mouse strains remains to be determined. The fact that skin grafts from perinatally castrated C57BL males enjoy a prolonged survival on isologous females suggests that endocrinological factors may be involved.

Clearly, genetic factors may not only be concerned with influencing immunologic reactivity, but they may also be able to influence immunogenicity.

REFERENCES

Billingham, R. E., W. K. Silvers, and D. B. Wilson. 1965. A second study on the H-Y transplantation antigen in mice. Roy. Soc. (London), Proc., B. 163:61–89.

Hildemann, W. H., and N. Cohen, 1967. Weak histoincompatibilities: emerging immunogenetic rules and generalizations, p. 13–20. *In* E. S. Curtoni, P. L. Mattiuz, and R. M. Tosi [ed.] Histocompatibility testing, 1967. Munksgaard, Copenhagen.

Strong and weak histocompatibility antigens. 1970. Transpl. Rev. III. Williams and Wilkins, Baltimore.

Chapter 4

Cellular and Subcellular Distribution and Nature of Transplantation Antigens

Investigations concerned with elucidating the location and chemical nature of the gene-determined substances that provoke transplantation immunity are important not only because they may afford some insight into the normal biological significance of histocompatibility genes, but also because of their clinical significance, i.e., the possibility of employing soluble, immunogenically active preparations clinically to induce tolerance of organ homografts (see Chapter 10).

Historically, the study of transplantation antigens has evolved from investigations of two quite distinct and apparently diametrically opposed findings with cell homogenates or extractives of various types:

1. The discovery that pretreatment of adult rat or mouse hosts with some of these preparations, derived from malignant or normal tissues that would normally be rejected, may specifically *promote* the growth of the graft, *prolonging* its survival. Although this phenomenon was reported as early as 1907 by Flexner and Jobling and was systematically studied in the 1930s and 1940s by Casey (who referred to it as the "XYZ" effect), it wasn't until the early 1950s that Kaliss and Snell at Bar Harbor demonstrated that it had an immunological basis. These investigators called the phenomenon "enhancement" and showed that it was put into effect by humoral isoantibodies produced in response to the inoculated extract or homogenate (see Chapter 7). In the mouse it was found that an essential requirement to obtain significant degrees of enhancement is that graft donor and host *must* differ at the H-2 locus; also, the effective antibodies are directed against the antigens determined by this locus in the homograft.

From observations such as these, the conclusion was drawn that in mice, enhancement—though apparently the opposite of transplantation immunity (it results from an immunity which *weakens* the normal resistance of animals to homografts)—is also the outcome of *active* immunization of a host by a substance closely related to, if not identical with, the H-2 antigen. Interest therefore centered upon the chemistry of the "enhancing substance," stimulated partly by the belief that it might afford a clinically applicable means of abrogating graft rejection and partly by the fact that it was a histocompatibility gene product.

2. On the basis of a) fifty years of unsuccessful attempts to incite resistance to tumor homografts by means of nonliving or disintegrated cells, and b) more recent findings that grafts of living skin or suspensions of living spleen cells completely lose their effectiveness in eliciting transplantation immunity after such moderate treatments as heating to 48.5°C for twenty minutes, repeated freezing and thawing, or drying from the frozen state, the frustrating view was sometimes expressed that the capacity to evoke sensitivity to homografts is the prerogative of *living* cells. Indeed, the work on enhancement appeared to lend support to this interpretation. Not until 1956 was this unsatisfactory state of affairs terminated and an element of mystique removed from transplantation immunology by Billingham, Brent, and Medawar. They found that, with H-2 locus-incompatible CBA and A mice, splenic cells which were totally disintegrated by ultrasonic irradiation in such media as buffered normal saline, isotonic saline, sucrose, or even distilled water retained their power to incite immunity to subsequent test skin homografts from the original donor strain.

Because appropriate, genetically defined experimental subjects in large numbers were readily available, the antigens determined by the H-2 and some other histocompatibility loci of the mouse have been those most thoroughly studied. However, important studies have also been made on the transplantation antigens of rats, guinea pigs, hamsters, and man.

Assay Procedures

Test systems developed to assay the antigens in cell homogenates and extracts fall into the following two categories.

In Vivo Tests

These include:

1. The time-honored determination of the capacity of a preparation to elicit transplantation immunity in a host, recognizable in terms of the accelerated destruction of a subsequent test skin homograft. It is an exacting test but somewhat cumbersome, and it requires a minimum of two weeks between administration of the antigen and histological evaluation of the test skin graft. Moreover, because of the flatness of the dose-response curve, this test is not very suitable for quantitation.

2. Determination of the capacity of high dosage inocula of subcellular antigenic material, either alone or in combination with immunosuppressive agents, to prolong the lives of subsequent test tissue homografts as a consequence of the induction of specific immunological nonreactivity or tolerance (see Chapter 10). Although this procedure is currently too difficult and time consuming to afford a practical means of assaying transplantation antigens, it is of some theoretical importance since it is the *only* one available for testing for the presence of *all* the disparate antigenic determinants in an extract that were present in the living donor tissue from which the extract was prepared.

3. Determination of the capacity of extracts, administered with or without adjuvants, to enhance the growth of appropriate test tumor homografts, or to incite the production of isoantibodies detectable serologically in terms of their capacity to react in vitro with erythrocytes or leucocytes.

4. Inoculation of the material into the skins of appropriate animals to determine its capacity to incite various types of delayed cutaneous inflammatory hypersensitivity reactions (see Chapter 8). For example, guinea pigs, hamsters, and certain other species which have been sensitized by means of living tissue homografts develop delayed, tuberculin-type, cutaneous hypersensitivity responses, known as "direct hypersensitivity reactions," if challenged intradermally with living cells or antigenic extracts prepared from the same donor strain. These reactions are fairly sensitive in terms of the amount of material that will incite a significant level of response.

In all the various in vivo assays so far described, the immunogenicity of an antigenic preparation may be greatly influenced by the presence of impurities which may exert an adjuvant-like action. Indeed, with some tests, the antigenicity of a preparation may deliberately be enhanced by addition of adjuvants and by selection of a particular route of inoculation into a host.

In Vitro Tests for Activity

This category of assays comprises tests for specific activity where the substances under consideration do not have to be in an immunogenic form. Putative antigenic material is assayed for its capacity to *inhibit* specific definable serological reactions such as hemagglutination or hemolysis in the mouse and other species in which the specificities determined by the major histocompatibility locus, such as the H-2, are expressed on erythrocytes. Since *all* the important histocompatibility antigens are strongly represented on leukocytes, antigenic material can also be assayed in terms of its capacity to inhibit agglutination of these cells by appropriate defined antisera or to inhibit their lysis when complement is added. Cytolysis of susceptible lymphoid cell suspensions and its inhibition can be followed by phase contrast microscopy, by the uptake of vital dyes such as trypan blue by killed cells, or by measurement of the release of isotope markers such as C^{14}, Cr^{51}, or P^{32} from previously labeled "target" cells. Methods depending upon determination of chromium release are particularly favorable because of their convenience and apparent objectivity.

Finally, recent preliminary studies by Manson and Simmons suggest that the response of normal lymphocytes, cultured in vitro for a few days, to antigenic extracts of homologous cells may furnish the basis of another useful assay system. This response is reflected by an increase in DNA synthesis and the development of homograft sensitivity which can be detected by a method developed by Dr. Herman Friedman (see page 117).

Although in vivo immunogenicity tests are essential to assess the usefulness of the product of extraction procedures and to relate its immunogenic properties to those of the intact cells from which it is derived, the utilization of in vitro tests is virtually obligatory to monitor the purification of a substance from a crude initial homogenate or extract. In vitro inhibition tests can be swiftly performed, are relatively free from interference by impurities, exhibit a direct dose-response relationship, and are sensitive and capable of yielding reproducible results.

Although it is generally agreed that the antigenic specificities measured by the various methods outlined are indistinguishable, the requirements for activity are not necessarily identical in all tests. For example, extraction procedures that separate antigenic determinants from their normal carrier macromolecules may totally abolish their ability to incite resistance to homografts (which, as we shall see, depends on a "cellular" immunity), while having no effect on their capacity to enhance the growth of test tumor homografts by evoking the formation of humoral antibodies. Possibly because of the small size of their constituent "particles" or fragments, or secondary changes resulting from extraction procedures, some cell fractions may be devoid of all immunogenic activity, yet still be capable of specifically inhibiting serological reactions in vitro, i.e., they behave as haptens.

To avoid confusion, we shall henceforth follow Dr. D. A. L. Davies and others in reserving the term "transplantation antigens" for preparations that can be shown to evoke heightened resistance to test skin grafts or to incite delayed cutaneous reactions, and we designate as "histocompatibility antigens" substances whose purification and antigenic specificity can only be followed by in vitro tests. The latter are *incomplete* antigens from the transplanter's viewpoint.

Distribution of Transplantation Antigens

With possibly a few qualifications (see Chapter 10), the full spectrum of antigenic specificities corresponding to an animal's endowment of histocompatibility genes seems to be expressed by all living *nucleate* cells of its body. This important general principle was first hinted at by observations that each of a wide variety of living tissue or "cellular" homografts will sensitize a host with respect to others of the same genetic origin. For example, pretreatment of a mouse with suspensions of leucocytes, or cells from different types of tumors, will cause it to reject skin grafts from the same alien donor strain in an accelerated manner (indicating at least a sharing of some important antigens by different tissues). This principle was further substantiated when it was found that animals made tolerant (see Chapter 10) by inoculation in early life with living homologous cells derived from one type of tissue usually were completely and specifically incapable of reacting against a variety of tissue and organ grafts from the donor of the tolerance-conferring stimulus or from another donor of similar genetic constitution.

Mammalian erythrocytes are anomalous in that, in all species tested, with the possible exception of man (see Chapter 2), they appear to be devoid of the capacity to provoke transplantation immunity, despite their expression of serologically detectable specificities determined by some histocompatibility loci, particularly the major ones (i.e., they lack transplantation antigens but possess histocompatibility antigens). The basis of this apparent shortcoming needs clarification since effective transplantation antigens are present on the nucleate erythrocytes of chickens, as evidenced by the capacity of these cells to induce tolerance of skin homografts. Explanations concerning the immunogenic inadequacy of mammalian red cells all take into account their high degree of specialization and assume that their progenitors do possess transplantation antigens. These cells may be ineffective vehicles for the transportation of antigens to immunologically reactive sites, or their antigenic determinants may be inadequately represented or attached to inappropriate protein or other carrier molecules. The inability of these cells to incite transplantation hypersensitivity in vivo is also paralleled by their inability to stimulate lymphocyte transformation in vitro.

The fact that most of the important transplantation antigens are strongly represented on leucocytes has greatly facilitated the development of histocompatibility typing procedures. The other formed elements of blood—platelets and thrombocytes—also appear to express transplantation antigens in both a serologically detectable form as well as a form that enables them to provoke weak levels of graft immunity. In mammals the capacity of whole blood to elicit transplantation immunity (or tolerance) resides exclusively in its leucocyte and (to a much lesser extent) its platelet components, being absent from red cells, lymph, plasma, and serum. Transplantation antigens have not been demonstrated in milk, urine, or the extracellular fluids obtainable by subjecting tissues such as skin to mechanical pressure.

The Ontogeny of Transplantation Antigens

As we shall see later (Chapter 12), the ontogeny of transplantation antigens is important for an understanding of the potential immunologic hazard to the fetus of mammalian gestation. That transplantation antigens are present well before birth was implicit in early observations that minced-up homologous embryos are highly effective in eliciting immunity against tumor or other tissue homografts. Unfortunately such findings failed to exclude the possibility of antigenic maturation of the grafted cells in their host.

More critical studies have minimized or obviated this possibility in various ways, including the following: (1) restriction of the time available for the embryonic cells to sensitize their hosts before test grafting; (2) evaluation of the capacity of embryonic cellular inocula to confer tolerance upon infant hosts whose "tolerance-responsiveness" is known to wane within a day or two of the time selected for injection of "antigen"; (3) preclusion of further differentiation of the embryonic cells under test by irradiation; and (4) determination of the ability of embryonic cell preparations to absorb a specific antibody, in some cases by employment of indirect fluorescent antibody procedures. Although very useful, the last method cannot reveal whether effective transplantation antigens are present.

Carefully designed grafting experiments have indicated the presence of transplantation antigens in chick embryos by the fourth day of embryonic life, and in mouse embryos by the eleventh day of gestation, and probably sooner. The independent demonstration by Drs. Simmons and Russell and by Dr. D. R. S. Kirby and his associates that tubal mouse eggs fail to develop if transferred beneath the renal capsules of specifically presensitized, instead of normal homologous, hosts strongly hinted that some histocompatibility specificities are present in mouse ova at the pretrophoblastic stage. Unfortunately, these experiments did not indicate whether the effective antigens were determined by the H-2 locus.

Drs. Heyner, Brinster, and Palm have been studying the influence of isoantibody and complement on the development of tubal mouse eggs to blastocysts in vitro. They report that, provided the zona pellucida has been removed enzymically, antiserum in the presence of complement causes the eggs to degenerate. However, specific H-2 cytotoxic antibodies fail to interfere with blastocyst formation, suggesting that if present at this stage of development, the H-2 determinant sites may be so sparsely distributed, or spatially oriented in such a manner, as to preclude a cytolytic effect. The authors tentatively conclude that the susceptibility of eggs to antiserum is due to the early expression of non-H-2 specificities.

In other experiments these workers freed two-cell stage mouse eggs of their zona pellucidas and treated them with specific H-2 and non-H-2 antibodies, followed by fluorescein-conjugated antimouse globulin. This gave only very marginal indications of the presence of H-2-determined specificities on the eggs. However, evidence of the presence of certain non-H-2 antigens was afforded by the bright fluorescence caused by three different antisera known to contain only non-H-2 antibodies.

Whether transplantation antigens are present on spermatozoa remains equivocal. Drs. Barth and Russell, using a fluorescent antibody technique capable of detecting H-2 specificities on lymphoid cells, were unable to detect these on sperms, nor could they detect the rather weak Y antigen by this method. However, Dr. Marta Vojtišková has recently reported findings obtained by means of a hemagglutination technique which indicate that at least some antigens determined by the $H\text{-}2^d$ allele of the mouse are expressed on sperm. Her experiments include results which appear to exonerate the unavoidable contamination by nonsperm cells (up to 10%) as being responsible for the hemagglutinin-absorption observed. In man, Fellous and Dausset have just reported that HL-A antigens are present on the surface of human spermatozoa.

Red cell antigens, capable of reacting with appropriate H-2 isoantisera, are not demonstrable in newborn mice though these cells become fully agglutinable within a few days.

Extraction of Transplantation Antigens from Living Cells

Immunogenically active, insoluble, subcellular material is obtainable from both normal and malignant tissue cells of intact animals and from cells propagated in vitro by a variety of procedures including: (1) disruption of the cells by ultrasonic irradiation (preferably at relatively low frequencies); (2) ultrarapid release from high pressures; (3) freezing and thawing; and (4) direct homogenization. Active material is also recoverable from tumor-induced ascitic fluid and from media in which cells have been cultured in vitro. The initial fractionation of the crude homogenates or other starting subcellular material is accomplished by differential centrifugation and/or density gradient centrifugation. In mice and all other species so far studied, the transplantation antigens, of which there may only be a small number of molecules per cell, appear to be structurally associated with insoluble lipoprotein material of the plasma membranes. However, at present the possibility cannot be excluded that some of the activity resides upon internal membranous structures of cells such as lysosomes. Evaluation of the significance of reports that transplantation antigens are associated with particular intracellular organelles must take into consideration possible contamination by fragments of plasma membranes. It may be noted that the association of transplantation antigens with plasma membranes has long been evidenced by the successful use of a variety of cell types in suspension for serological studies with isoantibodies and, more recently, by findings with fluorescent-antibody techniques.

Solubilization of the antigens from the crude, virtually insoluble, lipoprotein membranous preparations is an essential step for their further purification and characterization. It has been achieved, with variable degrees of success, by treatment of membrane preparations with detergents, organic solvents such as butanol, ultrasonication in aqueous media, and autolysis or digestion with various proteolytic enzymes. None of these methods seems capable of effecting the solution of all the antigenic material present, and their products vary considerably in their properties, making it difficult to collate findings from different laboratories.

Drs. Kandutsch and Stimpfling have used a nonionic detergent, Triton X 100, to extract active material from particulate preparations of a strain specific murine sarcoma. The activity is associated with a lipoprotein which is soluble in dilute solutions of Triton and recognizable in terms of its capacity to cause "active enhancement," to incite hemagglutinin production, and to inhibit hemagglutination. Digestion of the Triton-soluble lipoprotein with snake venom converted it into a water-soluble form which displayed increased hemagglutination inhibitory activity but reduced ability to enhance or incite hemagglutinin production.

By treatment of lipoprotein material of microsomal origin with butanol, Drs. Manson and Palm of the Wistar Institute, Philadelphia, succeeded in liberating 40 to 75% of the H-2 and non-H-2 antigenic activity from murine tumor cells. The lipid content of the solubilized material was reduced as compared with that of the starting material. The solubilized material was present in a highly aggregated form with a molecular weight of approximately 6×10^6 and was highly immunogenic, being capable of: (1) evoking transplantation immunity when administered with adjuvant; (2) eliciting both a primary and a secondary antibody response; and (3) inhibiting both the leucoagglutinating and cytotoxic activity of appropriate defined antisera.

Nathenson and Davies successfully extracted soluble H-2 antigen and several non-H-2 antigens from crude lipoprotein fragments of mouse lymphoid tissue cells by autolytic digestion. However, solubilization of H-2 antigen from lipoprotein material of tumor cell origin required treatment with complex enzymes of the ficin, bromelin, and papain group. Gel filtration of the soluble antigen removed inactive molecular fractions, yielding fractions which, though active on the basis of cytotoxic inhibition tests, were still considered as grossly impure on the grounds that the active regions did not coincide with other measurements made of protein, carbohydrate, or hexoseamine. Serological studies of this material after its further purification on DEAE-substituted Sephadex (Dextran) or cellulose columns revealed that some of the non-H-2 antigens were not solubilized by autolysis and enzyme treatment and that H-2 antigens were separable from other mouse isoantigens such as H-6 and TL (thymus leukemia) by ion exchange chromatography. Chemical studies on the soluble antigens indicated that they were glycoproteins.

Working with two different inbred strains of guinea pigs, Dr. Barry Kahan and his associates found that exposure of various types of cells to ultrasound liberated water-soluble transplantation antigens. Following removal of debris and cellular membranes by centrifugation at 130,000 g, these workers established that the antigenic principle could be purified by gel filtration on Sephadex G-200, followed by discontinuous electrophoresis on a polyacrylamide gel, to yield a relatively homogeneous material which they considered to be a "true transplantation antigen" by all criteria.

This guinea pig tissue antigen was reported to be a homogeneous protein, having a molecular weight of 13,000 to 15,000 and without detectable lipid or carbohydrate. The amino acid composition was characteristic and reproducible. Of particular interest and potential significance was the evidence that distinct and consistently demonstrable differences existed in the content of certain amino acids in the antigens prepared from guinea pigs of the two different inbred strains, the remaining amino acids being present in closely similar amounts.

Although it is now well established that the antigenic specificities of all histocompatibility genes are associated in the same fraction of cell membranes, and that solubilization liberates most of the known antigenic determinants, we still don't know whether these specificities all reside on the same molecule and whether, after they're liberated, they are still organized in the manner in which they exist on the cell membranes.

Dr. D. A. L. Davies has produced some evidence that the antigenic specificities determined by strong histocompatibility loci are separable by ion exchange chromatography and that some of them are present on single molecules. He treated antigenic material from an F_1 hybrid mouse with an isoantiserum directed against the tissue antigens of *one* of its parental strains and then isolated the antigen-antibody complex by gel filtration. Since this complex was found to contain the antigenic specificities of the other parent, he concluded that *both* antigenic phenotypes were present on a single species of molecule.

The important question whether at least the major antigenic specificities of solubilized and highly purified homogeneous material are determined by protein structure, rather than by subsidiary lipid or carbohydrate attachments, still awaits final resolution, though the former view is meeting with increasing favor.

The existence of wide quantitative variations in the amount of transplantation antigen present in different types of cells is indicated by the results of comparative studies of the capacity of crude homogenates of different tissues to absorb specific cytotoxic antibodies in mice. The highest concentration of H-2, and presumably Ag-B and HL-A, antigens exists in components of the reticuloendothelial system and the lowest concentrations in muscle, testis, and brain. On the other hand, some non-H-2 antigens have been reported in relatively high concentrations in the testis and the brain.

All authorities agree that the immunogenic potency of an extract is very much inferior to that of the living cells from which the extract is prepared. This cannot be ascribed to the capacity of living cellular homografts to proliferate after inoculation, since cells whose capacity to divide has been abrogated, by irradiation for example, are still immunogenically potent. This difference in sensitizing power between intact living cells and extracts is probably not due to large-scale loss of antigenic material during processing. The actual amount of antigen present on a living cell may in fact be exceedingly small. Making certain assumptions, Davies has estimated that the *entire* lymphoid tissue of a single adult mouse would yield only about 2 μg of H-2 antigen.

Although work in other species, particularly in man, has not yet progressed as far as the mouse work, the information available indicates that the specificities which are important in transplantation immunity are also associated with lipoprotein membranous material in cells and are closely similar in their general properties to those of the mouse. For example, solubilization studies have indicated that the HL-A system is the analogue of the H-2 system.

The Anomaly of the Liver

With respect to its transplantation antigens, liver seems to occupy a paradoxical position because, even though it is a very poor source of immunogens, its extracts are very effective specific absorbants of H-2 antibodies. A hint as to the basis of liver's immunogenic shortcoming was afforded by the finding that, in mice, when liver extracts are mixed with splenic extracts, the immunogenicity of the latter is abolished. Either liver contains enzymes that degrade antigenic activity or, as Manson and Palm have suggested, it contains a factor that prevents animals from reacting against transplantation antigens. It will be interesting to see whether any relationship exists between this peculiarity of liver extracts and the apparent immunosuppressive property of liver homografts in pigs (see Chapter 6).

Cross-Reactions

Various biologically or clinically important relationships have been established between certain antigens present in mammalian tissues and in microorganisms, and their investigation has provided important insights into the chemical nature of the determinants involved. Familiar examples are (1) the existence of shared or similar antigens of human and other erythrocytes and various microorganisms including Shigella, paratyphoid B, and pneumococci and (2) cross-reactivity between group A streptococci and various tissues, notably those of the heart, and the basement membranes of the renal glomeruli.

In the mouse, antigens from several microbial species, including Mycobacterium tuberculosis and Shigella dysenterieae, have been shown to exert an inhibitory effect on cytotoxic test systems, though the effect seems to be an overall one and is not directed against any particular H-2 specificity.

It is worth mentioning here that few attempts have thus far been made using either serological principles or accelerated homograft rejection to establish whether there is any overlap between the transplantation antigens of one species and those of another. Attempts to demonstrate overlap between the Y-chromosome antigens of rats and mice have been unsuccessful (see Chapter 3).

The interest of transplantation biologists in cross-reactivity was aroused by reports from Dr. Felix Rapaport and his associates that group A streptococci, Staphylococcus aureus, and S. albus are capable of inducing accelerated rejection of a high proportion of skin homografts in outbred guinea pigs, mice, rats, and rabbits. The activity of the streptococci as quasi transplantation antigens is localized to their membranes. Interest in this subject was recently heightened by the finding by Lange and Markowitz of a marked chemical similarity between murine H-2 antigens and those of group A streptococcal membranes, and by a report from Rapaport's group that group A streptococcal cell membrane antisera raised in rabbits, in addition to causing peremptory rejection of skin homografts in guinea pigs, also incited skin reactions characterized by polymorphonuclear leucocyte infiltrations in this species. This ability of the microorganisms, or rabbit antisera to their membranes, to cause accelerated destruction of skin homografts is limited to a certain proportion of their hosts, and is believed to be due to the segregation of the cross-reacting transplantation antigens in the outbred animals.

Interpretation of the significance of these apparent cross-reactivities will probably have to await further information on the chemical structure of transplantation antigens. Certainly repetition of the original experiments using isogenic strains of animals is absolutely essential to clarify the significance of the apparent segregation of reactivity observed in members of outbred stocks. Inbred stocks would also make it possible to conduct meaningful passive transfer experiments which are long overdue.

Concluding Remarks

There are many important unanswered questions about transplantation antigens. Are they constantly being released in either particulate or soluble form from cells and tissues in intact animals? The fact that cell-free membranous antigenic material is demonstrable in media in which cells have been grown sheds no light on this problem since it is not known whether the active material arises through cell death and lysis, or through release by intact cells. We don't know whether immunogenic subcellular material is released from homografts, though Dr. J. G. Hall's studies on the afferent lymph draining skin graft sites on the limbs of sheep have revealed that cellular debris passes along this route.

Snell has recently reviewed the comparative genetics of the H-2 locus of the mouse and has presented some interesting speculations concerning the possible biological significance of its polymorphism. He draws attention to the fact that the sharing of antigens between unrelated species (heterophil antigens), including mammals and their pathogens, is not uncommon. Snell deals critically with the hypothesis that such antigens might be of selective advantage to the parasite since the host would be unable to mount an immunological reaction against them because of *molecular mimicry*. Another possibility he considers is that, since transplantation antigens are probably important components of the cell membrane, and viral pathogens must penetrate this barrier to become established and survive, polymorphism at the H-2 locus may afford a protective mechanism which in some way increases the difficulty of viral penetration. Snell suggests that "different H-2 alleles are like different locks on different doors, which increase the difficulty of the burglar in gaining entrance." Consistent with this interpretation are a number of studies which indicate that H-2 genotype can influence viral oncogenesis, i.e., with any given oncogenic agent, certain H-2 alleles predispose to the oncogenic process while other alleles predispose to resistance. Moreover, the favorable allele seems to depend on the viral agent so that a rather intimate relationship between viral structure and membrane structure is suggested.

That transplantation antigens are important can scarcely be doubted from their presence in *all* vertebrate species so far tested, and from their faithful conservation by cells grown for prolonged periods in tissue culture and by malignant cells propagated for long periods in hosts that develop definite though ineffective levels of resistance against them.

In conclusion, we can only agree with Lilly and Nathenson that "we still don't know whether histocompatibility antigens are molecules that fulfill an important physiological or structural role in the cell; whether their antigenic properties, when placed in an alien, unnatural milieu are purely fortuitous; or whether their immunologic individuality reflects their primary function."

REFERENCES

Billingham, R. E., L. Brent, and P. B. Medawar. 1956. The antigenic stimulus in transplantation immunity. Nature 178:514–519.

Davies, D. A. L. 1968. Transplantation antigens, p. 618–634. *In* F. T. Rapaport and J. Dausset [ed.] Human transplantation. Grune and Stratton, New York.

Kahan, B. D., and R. A. Reisfeld. 1969. Transplantation antigens. Science 164:514–521.

Cross-reacting antigens and neoantigens. 1967. John J. Trentin [ed.] Williams and Wilkins, Baltimore.

Rapaport, F. T., A. S. Markowitz, and R. T. McCluskey. 1960. The bacterial induction of homograft sensitivity. III. The effects of group A streptococcal membrane antisera. J. Exp. Med. 178:514–519.

Snell, G. D. 1968. The H-2 locus of the mouse: observations and speculations concerning its comparative genetics and its polymorphism. Folia Biol. (Praha) 14:335–358.

Chapter 5

Immunologically Privileged Sites

Both malignant and normal tissues from fetal and adult donors have repeatedly been transplanted to anatomically unnatural sites in the body, i.e., grafted *heterotopically,* for a wide variety of reasons. These include: (1) technical convenience; (2) the ease with which a graft in a particular site can be palpated, measured, or visualized, directly without recourse to surgery, to enable its fate to be followed; (3) the study of tissue interactions at the morphogenetic level; (4) determination of the merits of various host sites to sustain various types of grafts; and (5) to appraise the roles of some of the variables in transplantation immunity. Homografts of skin and other tissues have deliberately been transplanted to regions of the body with major anatomic peculiarities, e.g., to the brain, which lacks a lymphatic drainage system, and to the anterior chamber of the eye or the substantia propria of the cornea in which, as in vitro, grafts may be maintained in a viable condition without penetration by blood vessels.

On the basis of this work, a considerable body of evidence, much of it of an empirical nature, has been accumulated attesting to the existence of "immunologically privileged" or favored sites in the body in which grafts of living tissues of alien origin may long be accepted by the host, apparently exempted from immunologically procured rejection.

The Anterior Chamber of the Eye

Most familiar of the favored sites is the anterior chamber of the eye because of the extensive use which has been made of it for tumor transplantation and the abundance of reports indicating that it affords a privileged site for homografts and even for heterografts. From a purely technical point of view, transplantation of small pieces of tissue into the anterior chamber is a simple and rapid procedure. If the grafts are deliberately located near the highly vascular iris, they acquire a blood supply fairly rapidly. Grafts which, because of their position, fail to establish vascular connections with their host may enjoy a more-or-less tissue culture-like, free-floating existence, sustained by the aqueous humor. A high proportion of initial "takes," characterized by continued survival and biological activity in their new milieu, have been reported for grafts of tumors, thyroid, ovary, lung, kidney, salivary gland, and skin in the anterior chamber.

Extensive studies by the late Professor Harry Greene of Yale University indicated that a high degree of success could attend the transplantation of both homografts and heterografts of malignant tissues and certain types of embryonic tissues to this site. Markee transplanted homografts of endometrial tissue to the anterior chambers of large numbers of guinea pigs, rabbits, and monkeys. He reported that the grafts rapidly acquired a blood supply and displayed the same cyclical activity in this site as in the uterus in situ for periods of up to nineteen months.

In a careful analysis of the fate of thyroid grafts in outbred guinea pigs, Woodruff and Woodruff found that, whereas only 11% of thyroid homografts transplanted subcutaneously were successful at the end of a 32-day observation period, 78% of the homografts transplanted to the anterior chamber were vascularized and still viable after an average observation time of 105 days. Other workers have presented evidence of the anomalous survival of adrenal homografts in the anterior chambers of mice and rats.

However, it must be noted that, despite these successes in maintaining homografts of various types in the anterior chamber, other workers have found that homograft survival is not significantly prolonged in this site. For example, Browning carried out a comparative study in mice of the fate of isografts and homografts of a variety of tissues and organs including skin, lung, and limb buds from fetal donors of various ages and from adult donors. He concluded that, whereas genetically compatible grafts displayed an initial phase of growth that was inversely related to the age of the donor, followed by indefinite survival, regression in the fourth week followed by death was the *invariable* fate of the homografts, irrespective of the age of their donor or whether they had entered a growth phase initially. In a subsequent study Browning and his associates came to essentially the same conclusion about the fate of homografts of adult or immature ovarian tissue transplanted intraocularly to adult mice. His findings do not exclude the possibility that the homografts he studied might have survived for a shorter time had they been transplanted to other sites.

The results of several recent studies on the survival of skin homografts in the anterior chambers of rabbits' and guinea pigs' eyes again indicate the need for further investigation of the immunologic status of this site. In the hands of some investigators, the majority of the grafts become vascularized and unquestionably survive for many weeks, whereas in the experience of others, immunologic rejection is the rule after no more than a slight prolongation of survival at the best.

Two important questions have been asked concerning skin homografts of various types transplanted to the anterior chamber: (1) are they effectively antigenic and (2) does the state of generally increased resistance evoked by an extraocular graft extend to the anterior chamber?

Evidence bearing upon the first question, in addition to that already considered, though by no means unequivocal, seems to indicate that grafts in the anterior chamber can elicit some degree of sensitivity to which they themselves may or may not succumb. Working with the Brown-Pearce rabbit carcinoma, Cheever and Morgan found that grafting to one eye did not prejudice the success of subsequent grafts of the same tumor to the other eye of a host rabbit. However, in Greene's experience, following homotransplantation of this tumor to the anterior chamber of one eye, both the contralateral anterior chamber and the testis were resistant to further grafts of the same tumor, indicating that grafts in the anterior chamber can induce immunity and that this is effective in the other anterior chamber. Some of the Woodruffs' findings on thyroid homografts in guinea pigs support this conclusion. When homologous thyroid tissue was transplanted to the anterior chambers of hosts whose *own* thyroids were intact, the grafts usually regressed, and the opposite anterior chamber became refractory to a further thyroid homograft from the original donor, despite thyroidectomy of the host in the meantime.

The second question can be answered unequivocally—sensitivity evoked by prior *extraocular* homografts does curtail the survival of subsequent transplants to the anterior chamber. Medawar transplanted tiny skin homografts to the anterior chambers of rabbits which had previously been specifically immunized by means of orthotopic skin grafts from the same donor. Histological examination of intraocular grafts that had been in residence for ten days revealed that those which had become attached to the iris and acquired a blood supply were destroyed, whereas those which had failed to acquire a blood supply survived. Since survival of the grafts was not dependent upon a vascular supply—indeed just the opposite was the case—Medawar interpreted these findings as affording strong disproof of the thesis that ischemia is the immediate cause of homograft breakdown.

The Woodruffs also found that prior subcutaneous transplantation of thyroid homografts to thyroidectomized host guinea pigs significantly reduced the chances of survival of subsequent homografts from the *same* donors to their hosts' anterior chambers. Medawar and Russell have obtained evidence that sensitization of a host *after* establishment of an endocrine homograft in the anterior chamber can also affect the well-being of the graft. They took adrenalectomized CBA mice which had been subsisting on intraocular homografts of A strain adrenal cortical tissue for two weeks and actively immunized them by intraperitoneal inoculation of A strain spleen cells. This caused the deaths of about 50% of the subjects from adrenal deficiency. Although the remainder of the subjects survived for at least fourteen days after the injection of the immunizing cells, they displayed unmistakable signs of adrenal deficiency, and their grafts were disorganized histologically and no longer vascularized.

The Cornea

In man the high proportion of successes that attend the use of corneal homografts to achieve a permanent and clinically successful repair of certain corneal lesions is in marked contrast to the situation with skin and other tissues. This apparent exemption of the corneal homograft from rejection has focused attention not only upon corneal tissue, *qua homograft,* but upon the intact cornea as a graft site that might have peculiar properties. Ophthalmic surgeons agree that, as long as penetrating or full-thickness corneal homografts are transplanted to avascular host corneas, the majority will remain clear. However, when the host sites comprise vascularized corneas, the percentage of grafts that remain transparent is greatly reduced. After a time interval which may vary over wide limits, a sudden dilatation of corneal vessels may be closely followed by opacification of the hitherto transparent graft. This delayed clouding, known as the *maladie du greffon* by French workers, has been equated to the homograft reaction as it affects other tissues.

Among the possible explanations put forward to account for the anomalous success of corneal homografts are the following:

1. The "dosage" of foreign corneal tissue used in keratoplasty may be so small as to be ineffective in immunizing the host strongly enough to cause breakdown of the graft. The fact that the epithelium of a corneal transplant is normally lost nonspecifically and rapidly replaced by the migratory activity of epithelial cells of *host* origin lends credence to this possibility.
2. Unlike skin and nearly all other tissues, cornea is antigenically ineffective, being incapable of eliciting an immune reaction.
3. Corneal grafts are in a privileged site which prevents them from eliciting an immune response even if they could succumb to it.
4. Corneal homografts, being unvascularized, cannot succumb to an immune reaction even if they can initiate one.

We will now consider the experimental evidence, forthcoming mainly from work carried out on rabbits, that helps to discriminate between these possibilities. So far as explanation 2 is concerned, it has been shown that, if thin homografts of corneal tissue are transplanted to extensive vascular beds prepared in skin, they are not long tolerated by their hosts. This is so despite the facts that they heal in well, they become vascularized, and their epithelium proliferates and begins to migrate centrifugally over the wound surface. They succumb to a reaction which resembles that which takes place in skin homografts similarly transplanted. Furthermore, animals which have rejected heterotopic corneal homografts become so affected as to accelerate the destruction of further heterotopic corneal grafts, or even skin grafts, from the same donors. These findings demonstrate that vascularized corneal grafts are capable of immunizing their hosts just as skin homografts do, i.e., corneal tissue *is* antigenically effective. So far as explanation 3 is concerned, it has been shown that, if minute skin homografts are tucked into small horizontal pockets prepared in the intact avascular corneal stromas of rabbits which had previously been immunized against their donor's skin, the grafts long outlive skin grafts transplanted on the same occasion to the recipients' chests, *provided that the intracorneal grafts remain unvascularized.* In those cases in which the grafts were located near to the periphery of the cornea, vessels from the limbus grew out and penetrated the grafts which promptly broke down. From this it may be inferred that tissue transplantation immunity is ineffective within the substance of the cornea so long as it remains avascular.

Further evidence in support of this interpretation was provided by Maumenee. He found that if rabbits received concomitant orthotopic corneal homografts and subcutaneous grafts of skin from the same donors, instead of remaining clear, the corneal grafts became inflamed and opaque within two to four weeks. The opacity closely resembled that seen in the delayed clouding of human grafts. He emphasized that vascularization of the host cornea is essential for this type of delayed opacification. Histological studies revealed that corneal grafts which become clouded develop lesions in their endothelium with resultant edema of the stroma. This is followed by a marked leucocytic infiltration associated with the invasion of the graft by blood vessels.

In both rabbits and man there is evidence of a progressive loss of vulnerability of corneal homografts to delayed opacification with time which may well be due to the occurrence of a slow, insidious replacement of donor stromal cells, or keratocytes, by host cells.

It may be concluded, therefore, that cornea is not an immunologically privileged tissue, but a tissue in a position that is immunologically privileged by virtue of its avascular status. The question of whether homografts transplanted to the avascular cornea can themselves provoke immunity is thus of no clinical importance, since any such immunity would be quite ineffective. Both clinical and experimental evidence suggests that orthotopic corneal grafts are perfectly capable of inciting an effective host response if they happen to become vascularized.

The Brain

It has repeatedly been shown, since the work of Shirai in 1921, that homografts and frequently heterografts of malignant tumors and homografts of embryonic tissues will often grow actively in the brains of adult hosts, whereas similar grafts transplanted subcutaneously or intramuscularly undergo rapid destruction. One essential condition for the survival of foreign grafts in the brain, insisted upon by Murphy and Sturm, who carried out an extensive study of this graft site, was that they must lie wholly within the substance of the cerebral cortex and not make contact with the ependymal lining of the ventricles.

However, as with the anterior chamber, not all investigators have found the brain to accept foreign grafts. For example, Lance has recently reported that intracranial thyroid homografts in adult thyroidectomized dogs failed to function, except perhaps evanescently and, on the basis of histological studies of biopsy specimens, gave evidence of only a very trivial prolongation at best. Moreover, such grafts induced a state of generalized transplantation immunity, revealed by accelerated rejection of donor skin grafts.

As a graft site, the anatomically distinctive feature of the brain is, of course, the absence of a lymphatic drainage. This has generally been thought somehow to underlie the longevity of grafts in this site, i.e., the brain fails to provide the *afferent* pathway of the immunologic reflex.

As with the anterior chamber, an important question pertaining to grafts in the brain is whether they will survive transplantation to presensitized hosts. To this Medawar obtained a negative answer. Skin grafts transplanted to the brains of rabbits previously sensitized by means of orthotopically transplanted skin from the same donors were found to be totally destroyed within ten days. This led to the conclusion that, although the presence of a lymphatic drainage may be necessary for immunity to be called into being, it is not necessary for its fulfillment.

The Cheek Pouch of the Syrian Hamster

Syrian hamsters have paired, backward prolongations of their cheek cavities running beneath the skin of their shoulder regions. They are richly vascularized and lined by a continuation of the hairless mucous membrane of the buccal cavity. Although, when empty and relaxed, the pouches are about 3 to 5 cm long and 1 cm wide, these "storage organs" can be distended by food to more than twice this size (Fig. 5.1). A very loosely

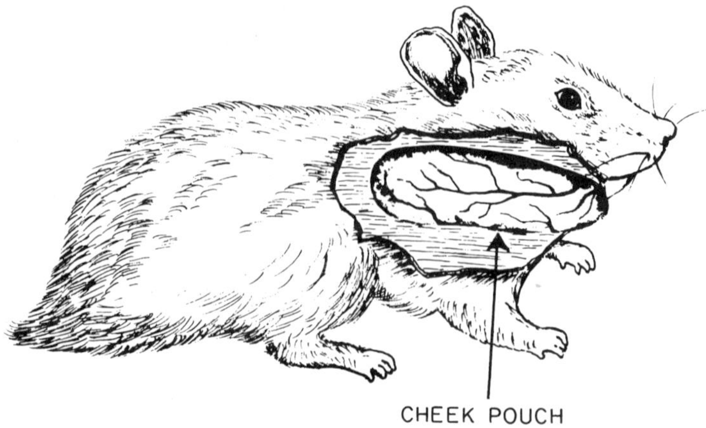

Fig. 5.1. A hamster in which skin has been excised from right side of head and shoulder region to show the distended cheek pouch. Note the abundant blood supply.

packed layer of highly elastic areolar connective tissue unites the wall of the cheek pouch to the overlying integument and to adjacent structures of the cheek, facilitating the complete eversion of the pouches from anesthetized animals (Fig. 5.2).

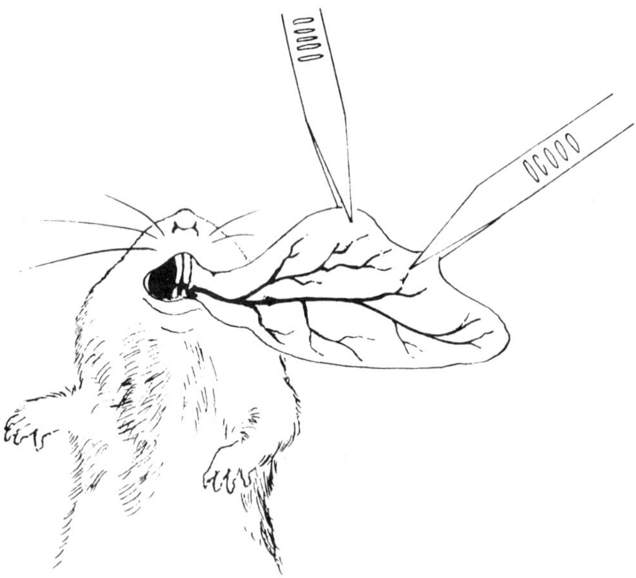

Fig. 5.2. The left cheek pouch is everted from the mouth of a hamster. Note the abundant blood vessels.

Everted, held under light tension, and transilluminated, the cheek pouch "skin" is useful for studies on the circulation because of its rich plexus of vessels and its semitransparency. Furthermore, as Dr. Lutz and his associates at Boston University first demonstrated, the connective tissue of the cheek pouch wall affords an exceedingly favorable milieu for study of implanted grafts of tumor tissues from other hamsters. Apart from sustaining the indefinite growth of homografts of normal and malignant tissues, this site will also allow the survival and frequently the growth of heterografts, usually of malignant tissues, from a wide range of donor species including frogs, mice, rabbits, and man for surprisingly long periods. With heterografts it is usually necessary to treat the host with an immunosuppressive agent such as cortisone to obtain impressive remissions of rejection. However, several neoplasms of murine origin will grow in the pouches of "unconditioned" hamsters.

The wealth of evidence on the continued survival and usually the proliferation of alien tissue grafts in the cheek pouch of normal, *untreated* hamsters constituted a prima facie case that this is an immunologically privileged site. Confirmation of this was forthcoming from studies involving comparison of the fates of skin homografts transplanted orthotopically, on the one hand, and implanted into the cheek pouch, on the other hand. In the former sites the grafts underwent prompt destruction, whereas in the latter sites the grafts acquired a good blood supply but survived indefinitely, being indistinguishable from isografts similarly transplanted.

However, like the other privileged sites we've considered so far in which the grafts became vascularized, the sanctuary afforded by the cheek pouch is also subject to the important qualification that it provides no protection against an independently elicited state of specific sensitivity in the host. Homografts are promptly destroyed if implanted into the pouches of previously sensitized animals, and the rejection of long-established grafts in the pouches of normal hosts is procurable at will simply by grafting the host orthotopically with skin from the original donor strain. These observations indicate that the hospitality of the cheek pouch to alien grafts is the consequence of some kind of break or incompleteness in the afferent pathway of the immunologic reflex. The consistent failure of all attempts to demonstrate a lymphatic drainage system in these organs affords a strong hint as to the basis of their privileged status as graft sites. Further information bearing upon this topic will be presented when we consider immunologically privileged tissues.

What is so convenient and interesting about the hamster's cheek pouch is that it retains its privileged status on transplantation. The cheek pouches can easily be removed from hamsters and cut open, and large sheets of "pouch skin" can be prepared from them. Transplanted as autografts or isografts to full-thickness beds prepared in the integument of the side of an animal's trunk, pouch skin heals in rapidly and retains its distinctive features, including its richly vascular status. More important, it retains its capacity to protect small or even relatively large *homografts* of ordinary skin carefully inlaid into very shallow beds prepared in such a way that a layer of pouch skin connective tissue lies beneath the homograft, separating it from host tissue below, and an annulus of intact pouch skin separates the homograft from its host peripherally (Fig. 5.3). With one

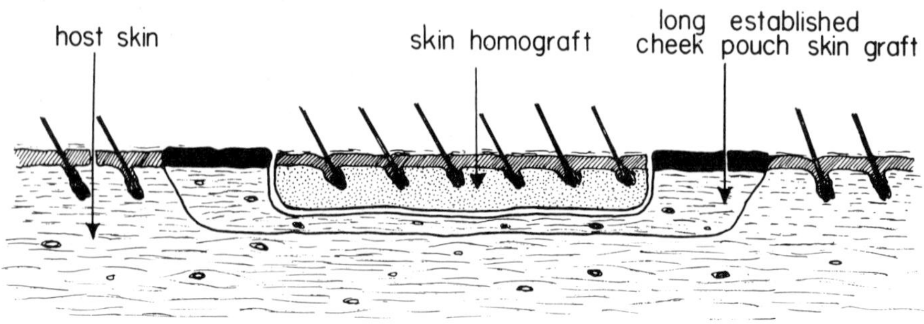

Fig. 5.3. This shows a long-established isograft of cheek pouch skin on the side of a hamster's trunk in which a homograft of ordinary skin has been inlaid. This graft is completely insulated from host tissue by intact connective tissue of the cheek pouch skin which protects it from the normal rejection process.

particular donor/host strain combination, whereas skin homografts transplanted to conventional beds survived for about eleven days, the majority of similar grafts inlaid into established pouch skin isografts lived very much longer. About 50% of them enjoyed virtually complete protection as indicated by their healthy appearance after one hundred days. Variability in the survival times of these sequestered grafts bore no relation to their sizes.

As with homografts implanted in the intact cheek pouch, these inlay homografts in the "transposed" privileged sites enjoyed no exemption from rejection if transplanted to specifically presensitized hosts. Furthermore, inlay homografts of long standing remained vulnerable to immunity elicited by *active* immunization of their hosts by means of parenteral injection of living lymphoid cells or orthotopic transplantation of skin from the original donor strain.

Pertinent to an understanding of the privileged status of these grafts is the following fact. Injection of a 2% solution of Patent Blue V dye via a fine gauge syringe needle, which affords a reliable means of revealing even the fine lymph vessels draining both intact skin and established autografts of conventional skin, fails to reveal *any* lymphatic connections between intrapouch skin homografts and the regional axillary, brachial, or cervical lymph nodes. If, as seems likely, the privileged sites afforded by ectopic isografts of pouch skin are due to absent or inadequate lymphatic connections with their hosts, the problem of accounting for the rejection of about 50% of the inlaid homografts remains.

The Testis

The testis is another site in which alien tumor grafts have been reported to thrive better than when transplanted intramuscularly or subcutaneously. One explanation of the as yet none-too-well established "special" property of this site focuses attention on the fact that there is an abnormally long lymphatic pathway between this organ and the nearest draining node located at the level of the kidney. However, a recent finding that small skin homografts transplanted near to the tips of rats' tails are rejected just as promptly as similar grafts placed upon the thorax suggests that the distance between the bed of a homograft and its nearest draining node is not an important factor in determining its expectation of survival.

Fat Pads

There is limited but nonetheless fairly convincing evidence that the mammary and other subcutaneous fat pads of mice also afford some degree of privilege in that the immunologic responses incited by small homografts implanted into them may be restricted. For example, Blair and Moretti have shown that the capacity of grafts of mammary tissue or skin from C57BL male mice to sensitize females with respect to the Y antigen (as evidenced by the survival of a subsequent male skin isograft placed orthotopically) is much less if they are implanted into a gland-free mammary fat pad than if they are transplanted subcutaneously. However, where stronger histoincompatibilities are involved, the privileged status of the fat pad was not demonstrable. Krohn, too, has observed that "pieces of mouse skin, equal in weight to ovarian grafts, may survive happily when transplanted into the fatty subcutaneous tissue of the chest wall." In his experiments H-2 incompatible grafts were used.

The Matrix of the Hair Follicle

If the epidermis is enzymically separated from the dermis of thin shavings of black guinea pigs' skin and transplanted to a very shallow "split-thickness" bed prepared in the white skin of an *isologous* host, the transplanted epidermal cells incorporate with the residual native host epithelial cells to produce a new epidermal system of *composite* origin. The evidence for this is that the donor pigment cells, or melanocytes, continue to function, producing intense pigmentation of the superficial epidermis and causing a significant number of the hairs which regenerate to be black in color. Pigmentation of both the superficial epidermis and of the hairs is valid evidence of melanocyte survival in these sites. When *homografts* of black epidermis from strain #13 donor guinea pigs are transplanted to shallow beds prepared in white skin of strain #2 hosts, it has been found that, whereas superficial pigmentation of the epidermis is only transient (disappearing within fourteen days or less after transplantation) as a consequence of the development of immunity by the host, black hairs are regenerated on the graft site. These black hairs continue to grow, retaining their pigmented status for upwards of forty to sixty days. This indicates that a level of sensitivity that is effective in destroying homologous melanocytes in the superficial epidermis is almost ineffective in prejudicing the well-being of homologous melanocytes that become incorporated in the hair matrices. The basis of this privilege against the fulfillment of an extant state of sensitivity is not known. It is tempting to ascribe it to failure of the melanocytes concerned to make their presence known and attract the presumed cellular effectors of transplantation immunity which circulate in the capillary tufts located in the papillae of the hair follicles.

An Artificial Immunologically Privileged Site in the Guinea Pig

More direct evidence as to the importance of a regional lymphatic drainage system for the development of immunity to skin and other solid tissue homografts has been forthcoming from Barker and Billingham's successful creation of a privileged site in guinea pig's trunk skin. Graft beds were prepared in circular, almost isolated, skin flaps raised on the sides of guinea pigs' trunks in such a manner that the *only* residual connection between the flap and the animal of which it was once a part was an intact vascular "umbilical cord" in which a lymphatic connection with the host could be retained or abolished at will. The wounds were surgically closed beneath the flaps and the latter housed in protective plastic capsules fixed to the underlying trunk skin (Fig. 5.4).

In the absence of demonstrable lymphatic continuity between the flap and the host, skin homografts fitted orthotopically into beds prepared in the skin flaps were not rejected so long as the flaps remained viable (twenty to fifty-seven days). Control skin homografts transplanted to similar beds prepared in *intact* trunk skin were invariably rejected within eight to ten days. When steps had been taken to preserve a lymphatic drainage in the

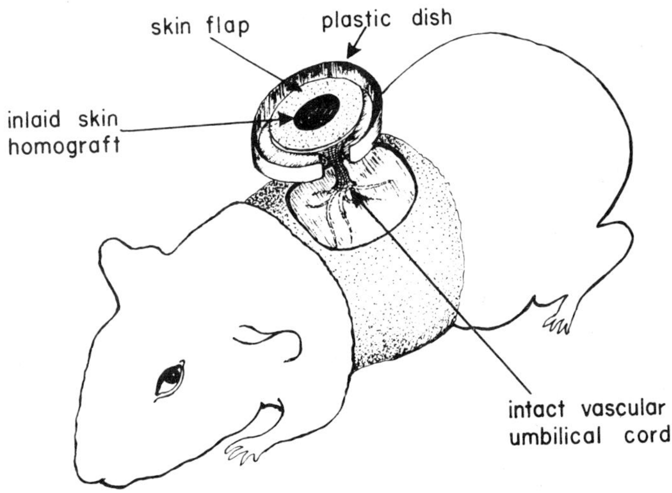

Fig. 5.4. A freshly prepared isolated skin flap with its vascular "umbilical cord" and inlaid skin homograft. After closure of the skin defect with sutures, the plastic dish housing the flap is glued to the underlying skin of the animal. (After Barker, C. F. and R. E. Billingham, 1968. J. Exp. Med. 128:197.)

host flaps, intraflap homografts were rejected in the usual manner. Hosts that bore healthy intraflap homografts of long standing gave no indication of being sensitized, as evidenced by their failure to reject orthotopically placed skin homografts from the original donor strain in an accelerated manner. However, intraflap skin homografts were rejected if: (1) the hosts had been presensitized; (2) a skin homograft was transplanted to a conventional bed at the same time that a similar alien graft was placed in a flap; (3) the lymphatic drainage was restored to a flap by reimplantation of the latter to an appropriate vascular bed; or (4) a host bearing a healthy intraflap homograft was immunized adoptively (see Chapter 8).

Conclusion about Privileged Sites

Although it seems well established that the various privileged sites described do possess properties that distinguish them from most other sites to which homografts are transplanted, it cannot be denied that a disturbing degree of variability seems to attend the capacity of most of them to extend the lives of foreign grafts. Further investigations are necessary to clarify the situation as it now stands. Most of the evidence bearing upon the immunological peculiarities of these sites rests upon studies in which animals of outbred stocks were used; hence the "average" genetic disparity between homograft and host probably varied widely from one investigation to another. Furthermore, different tissues, endocrine-versus-nonendocrine, normal-versus-malignant, fetal-versus-adult, have been employed for a variety of purposes. These tissues, as we shall see, do vary in their genetic requirements for survival, particularly in situations where differences at major histocompatibility loci are not involved. Further studies on privileged sites must take cognizance of these considerations. One thing at least is certain—the findings already obtained from work on privileged sites have yielded important information on physiological aspects of the homograft reaction.

REFERENCES

Billingham, R. E., and W. K. Silvers [ed.] 1961. Transplantation of tissues and cells. Wistar Institute Press, Philadelphia.

Billingham, R. E., and W. K. Silvers. 1962. Studies on pouch skin homografts in the syrian hamster, p. 90–108. *In* G. E. W. Wolstenholme and M. P. Cameron [ed.] Ciba foundation symposium on transplantation. Little, Brown and Co., Boston.

Billingham, R. E., and W. K. Silvers. 1963. Skin transplants and the hamster. Sci. Amer. (January), 118–127.

Billingham, R. E. 1970. Transplantation as evoked by skin homografts and as expressed in intact skin. *In* Advances in biology of skin XI. Appleton-Century-Crofts, New York.

Medawar, P. B. 1948. Immunity to homologous grafted skin III. The fate of skin homografts transplanted to the brain, to subcutaneous tissue, and to the anterior chamber of the eye. Brit. J. Exp. Path. 29:58–69.

Russell, P. S., and A. P. Monaco. 1965. The biology of tissue transplantation. Little, Brown and Co., Boston.

Ryecroft, B. W. [ed.]. 1955. Corneal grafts. Butterworth and Co., London.

Ryecroft, B. W. 1965. Biological problems of the corneal graft. Brit. Med. Bull. 21:147–152.

Woodruff, M. F. A. 1960. The transplantation of tissues and organs. Charles C. Thomas, Springfield.

Chapter 6

Special Properties of Certain Tissue and Organ Homografts

Immunologically Privileged Tissues

There is no doubt that differences do exist in the capacity of different tissues to survive after homotransplantation. These disparities become more discernible and more significant in situations where compatibility at major loci prevails. Among the factors that may contribute to this variability are the following:

1. The degree of cellularity of the tissue concerned.
2. The nature and abundance of its intercellular matrix.
3. The degree of vascularity.
4. The amount of nonspecific necrosis that follows "free" transplantation.
5. The mitotic activity of the tissue after it has become revascularized.
6. Whether the original vasculature of the graft is reutilized, as appears to be the case in skin grafts, or whether the graft vessels degenerate and revascularization is accomplished by the ingrowth of new vessels (initially capillary sprouts, which differentiate) of host origin, as in the case of most tumor and endocrine tissue grafts.
7. The capacity of the tissue to stimulate activity (the stromal response) on the part of host fibroblasts and vascular elements necessary for the healing-in process.
8. The quantitative expression of transplantation antigens on the cell surfaces, and the extent to which these may or may not be masked by cell products, etc.

There are a few tissues and organs which merit special consideration because of their ability to survive homotransplantation for strikingly long periods, if not indefinitely. These will now be considered in relation to the evidence that bears upon their ability to violate the "laws of transplantation."

Cartilage

For homografts of living cartilage, survival for periods that must be reckoned in months or years is the rule rather than the exception in all species investigated. The use of cartilage homografts for reconstructive surgery in man is commonplace. The specific capacity of living chondrocytes to rapidly take up radioactively labeled sulphate and utilize it in the synthesis of sulphated mucopolysaccharides affords a simple, fast, and unequivocal means of establishing the viability of a cartilage graft. Application of this technique has revealed the survival of chondrocytes in cartilage homografts of more than eighteen years' standing in man.

Two by no means mutually exclusive hypotheses have been put forward to explain the consistent and striking longevity of cartilage homografts. According to the first, cartilage as a tissue is only very feebly antigenic because the cartilage cells themselves have this property. The second hypothesis maintains that chondrocytes are similar to cells of other types with respect to their synthesis and expression of transplantation antigens, but they are "quarantined" from entering into immunological interaction with their host by the unique physicochemical properties of the ground substance or matrix surrounding them. Protagonists of this hypothesis have compared the role of the matrix to that of a cell-impermeable Millipore filter membrane in a diffusion chamber which allows alien cells contained within it to thrive in the body cavity of a histoincompatible host (see Chapter 7).

Various lines of evidence indicate that the immunogenicity of cartilage homografts is extremely feeble. For example, they do not readily incite the hypertrophy and cytological changes in draining lymph nodes that follow homotransplantation of other tissues. Furthermore, it is not easy, even by repeated grafting of a host with cartilage homografts, to evoke a level of sensitivity that will bring about the second-set type of rejection of subsequent test skin grafts from the cartilage donor. Although quite a marked mononuclear cellular response is frequently observed in the bed of a cartilage homograft in a normal host, it is usually transient and fails to produce tissue destruction. If cartilage grafts are implanted into specifically presensitized hosts, i.e., animals which have already rejected skin grafts from the cartilage donor, significant numbers of infiltrating cells do gather around their periphery, and a limited amount of tissue resorption does occur. But the process is very slow and may never proceed to completion. Viable chondrocytes are demonstrable at the graft centers at all times, despite peripheral loss of metachromatic staining of the matrix and failure of the cells to take up ^{35}S peripherally.

By enzymatic digestion procedures, viable chondrocytes can be freed of their matrix and handled as "cellular" grafts. Following injection of these cells into muscle or other host sites, they rapidly reorganize and form matrix, much as they do when explanted in vitro. Several investigators have now studied the fate of cellular homografts of chondrocytes prepared from nasal septa of rabbits and injected into normal hosts. All are agreed that these cells survive and regenerate matrix. However, some workers found that no mononuclear host cell reaction has been demonstrable, while others have found that, after a few weeks, the cartilage formed by homologous chondrocyte suspensions is invariably surrounded by infiltrating cells, whereas that derived from autologous chondrocytes is not. These observations suggest that chondrocytes are antigenic.

In a recent study of the fate of suspensions of monodisperse chondrocytes, prepared from fetal limb bone cartilage, injected intramuscularly into the tongues of normal and specifically presensitized homologous rat hosts, Dr. Susan Heyner has found that in both Ag-B compatible and incompatible situations a strong cellular reaction develops against the reorganized, palpable, cartilaginous nodules. This results in the destruction of a high proprtion of them within about three to four weeks, despite evidence that the transplanted cells had probably invested themselves with a new matrix within twelve hours of transplantation. These and other observations show clearly that chondrocytes do possess effective transplantation antigens and indicate that very small homografts of cartilage derived from cell suspensions are susceptible to host attack.

Hamster Cheek Pouch Skin

In the previous chapter we considered the hamster's cheek pouch as a privileged site and saw that grafts of pouch skin transposed to a hamster's chest still retain the capacity to protect inlaid homografts of ordinary skin.

It has also been found that, if *homografts* of pouch skin are transplanted to recipient areas in the integument of hamster's trunks, most of them survive for at least twice as long as homografts of ordinary skin of similar or much smaller size. In fact, a significant proportion survive in a healthy, isograft-like condition for fifty to one hundred days. Some of these hitherto healthy-looking pouch skin homografts of long standing are eventually rejected. Sometimes this is the consequence of a rapid reaction of abrupt origin, ushered in by edema, intradermal hemorrhages, and epithelial weakness. With other long-accepted pouch skin homografts, however, rejection is a chronic, drawn-out process in which there is epithelial desquamation, minor ulcerative lesions with partial recovery, and progressive contracture of the graft.

These striking prolongations of survival of pouch skin homografts suggest that pouch skin itself constitutes an immunologically privileged tissue. Unlike homografts of ordinary skin, either they represent a very feeble and often ineffective source of transplantation antigens or they are abnormally resistant to a state of sensitivity directed against them. This second explanation is untenable in the light of the following observations:

1. Hamsters that have rejected homografts of ordinary skin promptly reject subsequent pouch skin homografts.
2. Hamsters that have rejected homografts of pouch skin promptly reject a second pouch skin homograft, whereas animals bearing cosmetically perfect, first-set pouch skin homografts of long standing invariably accept such grafts.
3. Long-accepted pouch skin homografts undergo rejection within a week or two if their hosts are injected with living splenic cells or leucocytes, or are grafted with skin from a member of the original donor strain. This shows that pouch skin homografts are fully susceptible to an extant state of sensitivity directed against them.

Since grafting and other experiments have established that the epidermal cell component of pouch skin expresses transplantation antigens in an effective manner, attention was focused upon the connective tissue component as being responsible for its privileged status. The prolonged survival of ordinary skin homografts inlaid into heterotopic pouch skin isografts (see page 72) lent considerable support to the thesis that the connective tissue moiety of pouch skin provides a protective barrier, interfering with the afferent pathway of the immunological reflex. Direct evidence in support of this hypothesis was forthcoming from the following experiment. Sheets of the rather slimy layer of areolar connective tissue, which lies beneath the tougher, compact dermis of pouch skin, were removed from freshly excised cheek pouches and spread over standard graft beds prepared on the sides of hamsters' chests. Small homografts of ear skin were then placed over the centers of these connective tissue grafts. Although the interposition of the latter did not prevent the ear skin grafts from acquiring a good blood supply, it did interfere with their ability to sensitize their hosts, as evidenced by the long survival times enjoyed by many of them. Viability on the part of the pouch skin connective tissue was not an essential prerequisite for its protective effect since repeated freezing and thawing under conditions known to be fatal for cells did not abolish its ability to protect overlay homografts of ordinary skin.

All the evidence currently available suggests that the privileged status of pouch skin turns upon the alymphatic status of its connective tissue.

Skin from Perinatal Donors

Whether homografts of tissues from fetal or very young donors can outlive their counterparts from adult donors is still largely an unresolved question having both biological and clinical significance. So far as skin is concerned, evidence from clinical studies is equivocal, and an early claim that, in rabbits, homografts of embryonic skin survive much longer than grafts of adult skin still awaits confirmation. However, in two species, Syrian hamsters and mice, skin from neonatal donors has been shown to possess very interesting immunological properties.

In hamsters, which have a very short gestation period of only sixteen days, it has been found that with three different donor/host strain combinations, the median survival times of skin homografts from near-term or neonatal donors are significantly longer than those of skin grafts from adult donors. For example, with the MHA $\longrightarrow$ CB combination in which the MST of adult grafts is 11.9 ± 0.7 days, that of grafts of neonatal skin is 21.6 ± 2.4 days. In mice, with donor/host combinations involving only weak histoincompatibility differences such as the Y factor in C57/BL mice, or alleles at the H-3 locus, these observations were made. A significant proportion of grafts from neonatal donors may survive indefinitely, generating luxuriant crops of fur, and long acceptance of such grafts frequently renders the hosts incapable of rejecting subsequent grafts of *adult* skin of the same genetic origin.

Wachtel and Silvers have recently extended this principle to grafts of neonatal and adult skin exchanged between mice of strains C3H and CBA which, though having the same alleles at the H-2 locus, differ at many non-H-2 loci. With the C3H $\longrightarrow$ CBA combination in which the MST of adult skin grafts is 16.0 ± 1.35 days, some skin homografts from neonatal donors survived for upwards of one hundred days. An interesting finding was that males proved to be much more accommodating hosts than females. For example, whereas only two of eleven female CBA's accepted neonatal C3H grafts for more than one hundred days, nine out of ten male hosts accepted their neonatal C3H grafts indefinitely. This sex difference in response is consonant with other evidence that female mice are more reactive in an immunologic sense than are males (see Chapter 3). All the male hosts that permanently accepted C3H neonatal skin grafts accepted subsequent grafts of *adult* C3H skin as well.

With the reverse donor/host combination, i.e., CBA $\longrightarrow$ C3H, the MST of adult skin grafts was shorter (12.1 ± 1.05 days) and that of skin grafts from neonatal donors was found to be similar. However, if the C3H hosts were exposed to various sublethal doses of whole-body X-irradiation *before* grafting, differences between the survival times of the two chronologically different types of grafts become apparent. For example, after the receipt of 300 R, the MST's of adult and neonatal C3H skin grafts were 17.2 ± 0.95 days and 26.2 ± 3.0 days, respectively.

There is no doubt that in these situations grafts of neonatal skin are more resistant to weak levels of specific sensitivity than those of adult skin.

Furthermore, in some situations neonatal skin grafts can actually transform some animals displaying sensitivity toward grafts of adult skin into tolerant animals. Likewise, when a panel of normal animals is exposed to neonatal skin homografts, some may respond by becoming tolerant whereas others may become sensitized. Clearly, where only weak histoincompatibilities prevail, the relationship between tolerance and immunity is a relatively labile one.

Many questions must be answered before the peculiar status of neonatal skin grafts can properly be explained. Are their component cells inferior to adult cells in an immunogenic sense? Does their behavior reflect possible "quarantining" properties of their immature connective tissue with its sparse cell population and abundance of matrix? Do living cells and/or their degradation products have to escape from neonatal grafts into their hosts to effect the tolerant state, or are the essential transactions between graft and host conducted peripherally? Is the spectacular rapidity with which neonatal grafts heal in and generate fur related in any way to the phenomena described above?

That peculiarities of the connective tissue of neonatal skin grafts may in some way be related to their tolerogenic properties is suggested by the observation that hamsters that have accepted heterotopic pouch skin homografts for upwards of fifty days are nearly always incapable of rejecting neonatal skin grafts from the same donor strain, though their capacity to reject homografts of adult skin is not demonstrably weakened.

Endocrine Tissues

The subject of endocrinology has long been associated with transplantation insofar as a classical criterion for endocrinological function of an organ has been to be able to restore the effects of removing it by replacing it in the host in a position away from its normal vascular and nervous connections. The foundations of this subject were laid at a time when transplantation immunology was in its infancy and inbred strains of animals were either unavailable or their value was unrecognized. From the earlier literature of endocrinology, one gains the impression that the rejection of grafts from alien donors was a rare event, or passed unnoticed. It is even possible to build a reasonable prima facie case for believing that endocrine grafts enjoy a special dispensation from the normal rigors of graft reaction, at least as they apply to orthotopic skin grafts and subcutaneously implanted tumor grafts. Indeed, many of the investigations on the fate of endocrine homografts which have been carried out in the past two decades lend support to this view. Some of these are presented below.

In experiments performed on members of a small closed, and therefore partially inbred, colony of albino rats, Billingham and Parkes compared the survival of orthotopic skin homografts with that of subcutaneously implanted ovarian homografts in ovariectomized females. The cyclical activity of the vaginal mucosa, as evidenced by vaginal smears, afforded evidence of the functional status of the endocrine grafts. It was found that a degree of immunogenetic disparity between donor and host that would lead to the rejection of skin homografts was only rarely sufficient to affect the continued functional activity of ovarian grafts. However such ovarian homografts failed to survive when they were implanted into rats that had *previously* received, and subsequently reacted vigorously against, skin homografts from the same donor. This suggested that, with the immunogenetic disparities present in the heterogeneous rat population under study, although the majority of the ovarian homografts were incapable of provoking effective levels of sensitivity, they were fully susceptible to sensitivity evoked by prior homografts of skin from the same donor. An incisive demonstration of the superior resistance of ovarian tissue to homotransplantation was forthcoming when skin and ovary were transplanted *concomitantly* to the same host. In every animal that rejected its skin graft, the ovarian graft lived longer, and those animals which took more than seventeen days to dismiss their skin grafts failed to destroy their ovarian grafts.

Essentially similar findings have been obtained by Kastin and Gittes. Working with a closed colony of hypophysectomized Sprague-Dawley rats, they transplanted two pituitary glands to the kidney on one day, followed by an orthotopic skin homograft on the next. Whereas the skin grafts were rejected within three weeks, the pituitary grafts continued to thrive, and animals bearing them grew better than their hypophysectomized, ungrafted controls. Similar disparities between the survival of homografts of skin, on the one hand, and of parathyroid grafts, on the other, have been observed in rats by Russell and Gittes.

Almost without exception the interesting results cited, and many others not discussed here, have been obtained with partially inbred populations of animals displaying variable and, in most instances, relatively minor degrees of histoincompatibility. When ovarian grafts were exchanged between rats of *different,* unrelated strains, the endocrine grafts were usually rejected very promptly. Evidently, then, a necessary condition for an ovarian graft to succeed where a skin graft would normally fail is that the immunogenetic disparity must fall below a certain limit.

Krohn and various colleagues at the University of Birmingham, England, made a very careful study of the fate of ovarian homografts, using a variety of inbred strains of mice. They found that, in every donor/host strain combination tested (most differed at the H-2 locus), irrespective of whether the endocrine tissue was transplanted subcutaneously or orthotopically, the grafts were destroyed before they had an opportunity to produce estrogen.

More revealing, however, were the results of two independent studies they carried out on apparently similar populations of (CBA × A) F_2 hybrid mice. Mice of one of these populations received orthotopic skin grafts from parental strain donors, and those of the other population (all females) were first ovariectomized and then given subcutaneous ovarian grafts from parental strain animals. The purpose of both experiments, of course, was to determine the number of alien transplantation antigens with respect to which the particular tissue from one parental strain confronted hosts of the other (see Chapter 1). A significantly higher proportion of F_2 mice accepted the endocrine grafts for upwards of one hundred days than accepted skin grafts for the same time. More important, the majority of animals which had long accepted ovarian homografts failed to reject subsequent skin grafts from the original donor strain.

Subsequently, a Swedish investigator, Dr. Owe Linder, working with strains of mice differing only with respect to relatively minor histocompatibility factors also found that ovarian homografts implanted subcutaneously into ovariectomized hosts were not only accepted, but also ultimately rendered their hosts incapable of rejecting skin grafts of the same genotype.

These results have been interpreted as indicative of a difference in immunogenic properties between grafts of skin and ovarian tissue and, more specifically, of the capacity of subcutaneously implanted ovarian tissue grafts to induce specific unresponsiveness in situations where only minor histoincompatibilities are involved.

In chickens, too, a similar phenomenon has been reported, again in situations where only weak histoincompatibilities are involved. Orthotopic ovarian homografts in castrated males often survive permanently and somehow "condition" their host so that skin grafts of the donor genotype are subsequently accepted. Moreover, according to Dr. A. G. Cock, subcutaneously implanted testicular grafts in ovariectomized females are able to overcome even greater histoincompatibilities.

As already pointed out, the incorporation and revascularization of a free graft with its bed seems to depend upon two factors: (1) the responsiveness of the host tissue to the presence of the graft and (2) the capacity of the graft to evoke a stromal response, which seems to be highly variable. For example, adrenal tissue is said to be a poor evoker of stromal responses, and the connective tissue of the subcutaneous space is ranked poor on the basis of its capacity for a stromal response.

In attempting to interpret apparent differences between the behavior of skin homografts and endocrine tissues, the fact must not be overlooked that skin is nearly always grafted orthotopically to a site which facilitates very prompt vascularization (including reestablishment of the all-important lymphatic connections) and minimizes ischemic necrosis. This is not the case with subcutaneously implanted endocrine tissues. In fact, Krohn has suggested that the subcutaneous milieu may constitute a "semiprivileged" site, from the standpoint that the relatively avascular connective tissue capsules that develop around subcutaneous implants may help to protect them. Pertinent to this interpretation is Dr. Delphine Parrott's important observation that, in rats of the same closed stock used by Billingham and Parkes, whereas intrastrain ovarian transplants persisted in subcutaneous sites in ovariectomized females, they underwent destruction by a typical homograft reaction if transplanted orthotopically to the well-vascularized ovarian capsule.

One explanation for the recurring peculiarities of endocrine homografts is based on an extension of Halsted's Law, according to which such grafts can only succeed when there is an absolute deficiency of their secretions in the host, leading to their stimulation by trophins from the pituitary. Although most authorities are now agreed that the injection of trophins is of no value in prolonging the lives of endocrine homografts, there is convincing empirical evidence that they facilitate the initial establishment of both thyroid and ovarian grafts. Neither type of graft succeeds very well in hosts whose own homologues are intact. Removal of the host's organs probably removes a source of competition for the trophic hormones present in its blood stream.

The Phenomenon of Graft Adaptation

Before we leave the subject of endocrine homografts, it is appropriate to discuss the phenomenon of "graft adaptation." When the Woodruffs studied the fate of thyroid homografts in a heterogeneous population of guinea pigs, they found that, while 75% of the grafts became vascularized and lived indefinitely in the anterior chamber, they usually underwent rapid destruction (95% of them) if placed subfascially or subcutaneously. Furthermore, intraocular thyroid homografts gradually lost their initial susceptibility to sensitivity elicited by subcutaneous implants of thyroid tissue from the same donor. Subcutaneous grafts transplanted six months after an anterior chamber graft were destroyed, whereas the grafts in the eye showed no change. More interesting still was the observation that, in a high proportion of cases, when homografts that had been in residence in the anterior chamber for three to six months were removed and transferred to a subcutaneous site in the same host, they became vascularized and survived indefinitely. Obviously some kind of adaptation had taken place.

Woodruff has pointed out that thyroid homografts (and probably grafts of other endocrine tissues as well) in the anterior chamber normally undergo central necrosis, followed by regeneration from peripherally located surviving cells. As a consequence of this phoenix-like process, the stroma of such grafts is almost certainly eventually of *host* origin, and this may reduce the magnitude of the antigenic stimulus or alter the nature and/or magnitude of graft/host cellular interactions when such reconstructed grafts are transplanted. The possibility that adaptation might also occur at the cellular level has also been entertained.

Many examples could be cited of homografts which have been enabled, by a variety of artifices, to become established in alien hosts potentially capable of rejecting them. Subsequently, when host immunological competence has been restored, it has been observed that the established alien graft may continue to thrive even though the host may have received and rejected a second graft from the original donor strain. Although it is known that healing-in grafts are more susceptible to immune reactions than are well-established grafts, the anomalous survival of the primary grafts in such situations is sometimes attributed to adaptation.

In a recent study of Ag-B incompatible renal homografts maintained in rats by treatment with rabbit anti-rat thymocyte serum (Chapter 13), Guttman and his associates have produced evidence of a progressive reduction in graft immunogenicity with time. This evidence is based on attempts to immunize hosts adoptively against their renal grafts and to transfer renal homografts of long standing from treated to normal rats of the same host strain. Among various explanations, they suggest that this may be due, in part at least, to a loss of cells of donor hematopoietic tissue origin from the interstitial tissue of the grafted organs. The role of adventitious passenger cells in the sensitization of hosts against organ homografts is discussed in Chapter 8.

Tumor Homografts

As we've already seen, nearly all primary tumors and their derivatives propagated within the strain of origin faithfully obey the genetic laws of transplantation. Indeed, these laws were based on the results of tumor grafting experiments and only later were shown to apply to normal tissues. Very occasionally, however, a primary tumor is found that will grow in an alien host strain.

The survival of tumor homografts can be augmented by passaging recently established strain-specific tumors in homologous hosts whose capacity for immunologic response has been partially abrogated. As a result of this procedure, stable nonspecific tumor lines may result, proving lethal to most *normal* homologous hosts. This is generally agreed to be principally the outcome of selective pressures acting on a population of rapidly proliferating cells. Cells with the most rapid proliferative capacity are probably selected for; therefore, by the time the host has developed what would be an effective level of sensitivity for a normal tissue homograft, the tumor transplant will have managed to attain a size that puts it beyond the reach of immunological control. These variant clones of tumor cells are characterized by reduced surface complements of H-2 and other important transplantation antigens. They are, therefore, of diminished immunogenicity (another important contributory factor in the development of "transplantable" tumors). In no case, however, is this "antigenic simplification" complete. Such tumors always retain the essential characteristics of homografts in the sense that hosts can be specifically preimmunized against them, i.e., they do not completely lose their individual H-2 and other specificities.

The classic example of a nonspecific tumor is the familiar Ehrlich ascites tumor, one of the most malignant of all mouse tumors. Originating in a mouse of unknown genetic constitution, it has been maintained by mouse-to-mouse passage since 1896.

There is also evidence that certain types of transplantable tumor cells can produce substances such as sialomucin, which may simply "smother" the transplantation antigens on their surfaces or otherwise interfere with the activity of the effectors of transplantation immunity.

Skin Homografts from Patients with Malignant Disease

Transplantation antigens seem to be so firmly engrained into the texture of tissues that it's hard to conceive of any treatment of a host that could affect the antigenicity of his cells and tissues. Nevertheless, a hint that perhaps this is not utterly impossible comes from a fairly recent report from D. B. Amos and his associates at Duke University. They found that skin grafts transplanted from five out of six patients with breast cancer or rhabdomyosarcoma to totally unrelated normal subjects enjoyed greatly prolonged survivals—upwards of twenty days; four of them living for longer than thirty days. These survivals were documented by cytogenetic evidence of the persistence of donor cells. Microscopy of biopsy specimens from the grafts revealed extensive mononuclear cell infiltration but little damage to epidermal cells. So far no equivalent observation has been made with skin homografts from experimental animals afflicted by malignancies. However, it does appear to constitute another of those provocative exceptions that make transplantation immunology so fascinating.

Organ Transplants

The increasing attention now being devoted to the study of organ homografts in small experimental animals such as rabbits, rats, and most recently marmosets, in part facilitated by advances in the technique of microvascular surgery, has brought to light several anomalous phenomena which fall within the scope of this chapter.

Kidney Homografts

In the rat, it has been found that the intensity of an animal's response to a kidney homograft does not necessarily parallel its response to a skin homograft of the same genetic origin, especially when Ag-B compatibility prevails. For example, White and Hildemann found that, whereas skin homografts from Fischer donors to Ag-B compatible Lewis recipients are regularly rejected in an acute manner within twelve days, orthotopic renal homografts remain functionally active for up to forty-eight weeks. Indeed, Fischer kidney grafts even display prolonged survival in Lewis hosts which are subsequently challenged with and promptly reject Fischer skin grafts.

Liver Homografts

Although the survival times of Ag-B incompatible liver homografts in rats are comparable with those of grafts of skin, the results of extensive studies on liver homografts in dogs treated with azathioprine, conducted by Dr. Thomas Starzl and his group at the University of Colorado, hint that, at least in this species, these organs may fare somewhat better.

In the pig, as Dr. Roy Calne and co-workers of Cambridge, England, have shown, liver homografts have quite striking properties. While pigs reject homografts of skin, kidneys, or hearts in a perfectly conventional manner, rejection of orthotopic livers is usually a slow and remarkably mild process. These organs are accepted and sustain their hosts for periods of up to eighteen months in the absence of *any* immunosuppressive therapy. Even more striking is the observation that, if either skin, renal, or auxiliary cardiac homografts are transplanted simultaneously with a liver homograft from the same donor to the same host, their survival may be significantly prolonged, the protection of the kidney from rejection being especially impressive. This protective effect, which also results from auxiliary liver transplants, evidently does not require chronic exposure to the liver graft since it has been found that transient exposure of a host to an auxiliary liver graft for only twenty-four hours suffices to prolong the life of a donor specific renal graft. However, even in cases where liver grafts are allowed to persist, their protective effect is not complete. It is most effective for a liver homograft itself, and least effective for skin, with renal homografts enjoying an intermediate degree of protection.

The survival of these liver homografts is also influenced by the immunological state of the host. For example, some pigs which receive concomitant grafts of liver and skin from the same donor accept the former and reject the latter, whereas no privilege is enjoyed by liver homografts transplanted to pigs *presensitized* by donor skin or kidney tissue.

Among various facts and observations that may shed some light on the intriguing behavior of the porcine liver homograft are the following. Although pigs are not deficient in blood lymphocytes and lymphoid tissues, their afferent lymph contains very few lymphocytes; hence, no large-scale recirculation can take place from blood to lymph via the nodes (Chapter 8). In mice, as already mentioned (Chapter 4), the liver contains an agent capable of inactivating transplantation antigens extracted from lymphoid tissue or of nonspecifically blocking a host's response to them. Indeed, because of this, Barker and Corriere ingeniously investigated the possibility that the intact liver might be capable of inactivating transplantation antigens of renal origin in dogs if the venous effluent is diverted from kidney homografts into the hepatic portal vein instead of into the inferior vena cava. Although this artifice failed to prolong the lives of primary renal transplants, Fukuda and his colleagues have recently reported that it will abrogate the ability of dogs to reject second-set renal homografts in an accelerated manner—a rather provocative and inexplicable observation.

Although they have not entirely discarded other possibilities, Dr. Calne and his associates believe that, in pigs, liver homografts release histocompatibility antigens in a form that is particularly effective in inducing tolerance in adult hosts. Moreover, they have obtained a hint that a similar state of affairs may apply in rhesus monkeys.

Heart Transplants

Ever since Dr. Christiaan Barnard performed the first human heart transplant on Mr. Washkansky at the end of 1967, followed by his dramatic rehabilitation of Dr. Blaiberg with a donor heart, there has been speculation whether this organ may not be a particularly favorable one for transplantation. Its relatively simple structure and metabolic function, compared with the kidney and liver, have been cited as possible contributory factors to its postulated superiority. However, there is little experimental evidence to sustain this optimism. Few of the many dogs that have received orthotopic cardiac transplants have survived for as long as a year, and all longstanding cardiac homografts studied histologically have shown vascular lesions involving the coronary arteries which are indicative of low grade rejection processes at work. The cumulative results of 150 human cardiac transplants point in the same direction. However, it may be significant that neither in dogs nor in man were the grafts studied obtained from well-matched donors.

In rats Ag-B incompatible auxiliary hearts whose blood supplies are maintained by appropriate anastomoses to the inferior vena cava and abdominal aorta are normally rejected within nine to thirteen days. However, Barker and Billingham have recently found that, with the Ag-B compatible Lewis ⟶ Fischer combination, auxiliary heart transplants do significantly outlive skin homografts. In a more critical comparison of these two types of homografts, skin and auxiliary hearts were transplanted from (Fischer × Lewis) F_1 × Lewis backcross donors to Lewis hosts. While the majority of the skin grafts were rejected within fifteen days, most heart grafts from the same donors remained viable and displayed some contractile activity of their musculature for upwards of one hundred days. Indeed, judged in terms of their functional activity, i.e., the strength of their beat, it is estimated that by the fiftieth day of transplantation at least 75% of these grafts could have sustained life.

This work on cardiac homografts emphasizes the difficulty of making meaningful comparisons between the survival times of different tissues and organs and indicates that, in some circumstances, a considerable proportion of the alien cellular population of an organ may significantly outlive its "functional survival time" as judged in physiological terms.

Teeth

In the eighteenth century John Hunter transplanted a few erupted teeth as homografts in man for cosmetic reasons. The results were disappointing, no doubt in part because of the intervention of sepsis. Both clinically and experimentally it has been shown that, if developed teeth are removed from their sockets and immediately replaced, they become firmly reattached by regeneration of the periodontal membrane and fulfill a useful function. However it is not known whether viability of any of the cellular elements of the tooth is essential at the time of transplantation.

Autotransplantation of unerupted teeth is also technically feasible and has indeed proved clinically useful in some patients. Again, though, it has yet to be shown whether viability on the part of any of the cellular elements of the tooth is necessary to facilitate both the healing-in and subsequent eruption of the graft. There is also some evidence of clinical success with tooth germ *homografts*. Experimental studies on such grafts in rats indicate that, although strong histoincompatibilities preclude their acceptance, these appendages are much less stringent in their histocompatibility requirements than are skin grafts.

Clearly, there is a need for more critical studies on tooth homografts and especially on tooth germs at a very early stage of their development. Present evidence suggests that they belong to the homostatic category (see below).

Homostatic and Homovital Grafts

From the viewpoint of their clinical application, homografts can be divided into two categories:

1. *Homovital* grafts in which persistent viability of the original cell population is mandatory for the graft to fulfill a useful function. Grafts in this category include skin, kidneys, hearts, and indeed all organ grafts, as well as tissues of the lymphohematopoietic tissue system.
2. *Homostatic* grafts whose role is largely mechanical, such as blood vessel segments, bone, cartilage, tendons, and fascia, and in which viability is not esential even at the time of transplantation. The inert materials that form a relatively large proportion of these tissues provide an essential supporting framework or matrix which becomes repopulated by invading cells from the host. These grafts retain their physical properties sufficiently well to serve their physiological function for clinically useful time periods.

The long-term preservation of homostatic grafts is relatively simple—they may even be stored in the lyophilized state at room temperature. Provided that they have not been denatured, devitalized homostatic grafts retain their capacity to elicit the formation of isoantibodies, though they are incapable of evoking transplantation immunity.

The Orthotopic Skin Homograft

Because of the ease with which skin can be transplanted orthotopically and subsequently scored for its degree of epithelial survival, a great deal of our knowledge of the fundamental principles of transplantation immunology is based upon studies conducted with this tissue. For many years there was a tendency to regard the skin homograft as fully representative of homografts of normal solid tissues and organs in general, and to consider as exceptions those tissues whose immunological properties, or genetic requirements for success, differed from that of skin. However, as much of the evidence reviewed in this chapter has shown, this view is no longer tenable: the skin graft *itself* must be regarded as one of the most exacting of all homografts.

There is a considerable weight of empirical evidence that prolonging the life of a skin homograft represents a much more formidable problem than prolonging the life of organ homografts. Thanks to the increased emphasis being placed upon experimental organ transplantation it has become apparent that, in certain circumstances and particularly when donor and host are similar at a major histocompatibility locus, skin grafts provide an unduly pessimistic picture of the fate of homografts in general. This situation seems more likely to depend upon the mode or *site* of grafting than upon any intrinsic immunogenic properties of skin itself. This follows from the following facts: (1) skin grafts are usually very small in comparison to grafted hearts, kidneys, or livers and, consequently, provide a relatively small aggregate vascular endothelial surface with which host lymphocytes can interact; (2) there is no convincing evidence that suspensions of epidermal cells are more immunogenic than, say, those of lymphoid cells.

Among possible factors that may either singly or in combination account for the anomalous behavior of orthotopic skin homografts are:

1. Skin homografts bring their full antigenic potential to bear directly upon a *single* regional or draining node system via the intralymphatic route, irrespective of whether it is mediated by the passage of antigenic material or of appropriate, antigen-sensitive, small lymphocytes which have been immunologically "primed" peripherally. In other organ homografts, by contrast, in which vascular anastomoses are established at the time of grafting, their immunogenic potential is almost certainly brought to bear principally via the intravascular route. This route is known to be not very effective in eliciting cellular immunity, but it may be superior in eliciting humoral antibody responses which can interfere with the development or expression of cellular immunities, leading to the phenomenon of immunological enhancement (see Chapter 7).

2. Whenever an individual is exposed to a homograft, some of his antigen-sensitive cells will be committed along the pathway that leads to sensitization, whereas others will be inactivated or eliminated as a consequence of the induction of some degree of tolerance. The level of reactivity of the host against the graft will be the result of these two vectors. Skin grafts may be much less effective tolerance-inducers than organ grafts that require vascular anastomoses, especially since it is well established that tolerance is most readily produced by administering antigen via the intravenous route (Chapter 10).

3. The execution of all free skin grafts involves juxtaposition of two cut raw tissue surfaces. Consequently, considerable nonspecific inflammatory reactivity at the graft-host interface is an unavoidable complication which may play a role in mobilizing antigen-sensitive cells and will certainly be effective in attracting macrophages to the site. These cells, which are known to be present in large numbers in the lymph draining a graft bed, play an important intermediary role in processing some kinds of antigens and may also be important in the inductive phases of transplantation immunity. Steinmuller's observation that low dosages of homologous cells in suspension are more effective in sensitizing hosts when inoculated into freshly transplanted skin isografts than when introduced into intact skin is pertinent here.

4. Some degree of nonspecific ischemic necrosis is an unavoidable accompaniment of free skin grafting, though its extent is normally concealed by the extraordinary regenerative capacity of skin. Autolytic processes associated with this nonspecific necrosis during the healing-in phase may facilitate the release of antigenic material and/or material having an adjuvant-like action.

REFERENCES

See references cited for Chapter 5; also the following:

Billingham, R. E., and C. F. Barker. 1969. Recent developments in transplantation immunology, Parts I and II. Plast. Reconstr. Surg. 43:559–568 and 44:20–29.

Billingham, R. E., and W. K. Silvers. 1964. Studies on homografts of fetal and infant skin and further observations on the anomalous properties of pouch skin grafts in hamsters. Roy. Soc. (London), Proc., B. 161:168–190.

Hellström, K. E., and G. Möller. 1965. Immunological and immunogenetic aspects of tumor transplantation. Progress in allergy 9:158–245.

Krohn, P. L. 1965. Transplantation of endocrine organs. Brit. Med. Bull. 21:157–162.

Rapaport, F. T., and J. Dausset [ed]. 1968. Human transplantation. Grune and Stratton, New York.

Silvers, W. K. 1968. Studies on the induction of tolerance of the H-Y antigen in mice with neonatal skin grafts. J. Exp. Med. 128:69–83.

Chapter 7

The Mediators of Transplantation Immunity: I. The Role of Antibodies

When animals are exposed to solid or dissociated cellular homografts of malignant or normal tissues, a variety of humoral isoantibodies are formed. These have been identified as hemagglutinins, hemolysins, leukocyte agglutinins, and cytotoxins. Breeding and grafting tests have shown that the antigens responsible for the formation of these humoral antibodies are determined by histocompatibility genes. For example, in mice all the evidence suggests that there is a single class of isoantigens determined by the H-2 locus and that these antigens are shared by erythrocytes and tissue cells, manifesting themselves in serologic work as blood-group antigens and in transplantation studies as histocompatibility antigens. Indeed, as we have seen (Chapter 2), the capacity of transplantation antigens to evoke a humoral as well as a cellular response serves as the basis for tissue typing procedures.

The difficult question now to be considered is what role, if any, do these isoantibodies play in the rejection of homografts?

Because, initially, it seemed that the humoral antibody response to a homograft was very much delayed, reaching its peak only *after* destruction of the graft, this was cited as part of the evidence that humoral factors do not play a significant role in the rejection process. However, subsequent studies using more sensitive serological techniques showed that, with a variety of mouse tumor homografts, antibodies are demonstrable in the serum soon after grafting, from the fourth day onward, i.e., *prior* to the onset of any histological signs of homograft rejection. Moreover, contrary to previous belief, they reach their maximum titer at about the time graft destruction is complete.

In considering the role of isoantibodies in homograft rejection, it is important to distinguish between homografts of dissociated cells and those of solid tissues. Certainly, in the former case there is no doubt but that isoantisera can have devastating effects. Not only are dissociated viable cell suspensions of lymphoid tissues, bone marrow, leukemic tumors, and epidermis susceptible to the action of antibodies, in the presence of complement, in vitro, but resistance to cellular homografts of these tissues can also be transferred passively in vivo by means of serum. For example, baby mice or rats inoculated with homologous adult lymphoid tissues can be protected against runt disease (see Chapter 11) by inoculation of appropriate isoimmune sera, or even as a consequence of acquiring the antibodies passively from their mother principally during life in utero. In fact, the ability of isoantisera to prevent or mitigate the development of runt disease as a result of its specific, complement-mediated, cytotoxic effect greatly exceeds that of specifically sensitized lymph node cells. This finding is not too surprising inasmuch as one might expect that antibody molecules would be a more effective means of eradicating or inactivating a chimeric cell population than some kind of cell-bound effector mechanism.

The destructive effect which isoantiserum has on dissociated cell suspensions is also illustrated by its capacity to abolish the protective effect which homologous bone marrow cells have on lethally X-irradiated mice. Whereas mice that have been lethally irradiated can be rehabilitated by intravenous inoculation with homologous bone marrow cells, those treated in this fashion but which receive an additional intraperitoneal inoculation of isoantiserum directed against the bone marrow donor do not survive.

The evidence incriminating humoral factors as *major* contributors to the destruction of solid tissue homografts remains unsatisfactory. Indeed there are findings that tell heavily against this premise, favoring the view that, so far as the majority of types of solid tissue homografts are concerned, destruction is mediated by a cellular rather than a humoral immunity. At least in rats, it must be conceded that some success has attended attempts to abolish tolerance of long established skin homografts with isoantisera. However, this seems to be due to the capacity of the antisera to destroy cell chimerism, i.e., eliminate the persistence of antigen which is apparently required for maintaining tolerance, rather than its ability to act directly upon the skin homograft and destroy it. Evidence for this stems from the fact that such grafts rarely undergo acute rejection but persist for several weeks after the last injection of antiserum before they are sloughed. It should be noted, however, that a different situation does occur in ducks for, as Hašek and his associates in Prague have shown, passive transfer of very large amounts of hyperimmune isoantisera to tolerant hosts is followed by the development of overt lesions in established skin homografts within a few hours, and their total destruction within a day or two.

There are also reports that skin homograft rejection in rodents can sometimes be accelerated by appropriate treatment of the host with immune sera. The best results have usually been obtained by *local* injections near the graft, rather than by systemic injection, and by the employment of antisera from hyperimmunized animals. Moreover, antiserum treatment seems to be particularly effective when administered either just prior to or soon after homograft challenge, suggesting that healing-in grafts are particularly susceptible to its effect. Probably the best evidence for this stems from clinical observations that, if individuals receiving kidney transplants *already* possess antibodies directed against the leukocytes of the organ donor, as a consequence of prior blood transfusions or rejection of a previous renal graft, a hyperacute rejection of the kidney may occur within a matter of hours. Because of this, a meaningful prognosis for a kidney homograft can only be made on the basis of histocompatibility tests if no circulating antibodies are demonstrable in the recipient's serum reactive with the donor's leukocytes.

In discussing the role that humoral antibodies play in the rejection of homografts, one should not omit the classic experiments of the late Glenn Algire and his colleagues at the National Institutes of Health. They studied the fate of tiny homografts of fetal mouse lung, skin epithelium, etc., enclosed within diffusion chambers comprised of membranes perforated by pores of known diameter and inserted into the peritoneal cavities of host mice. If the latter were specifically sensitized, then the target homografts underwent destruction only if the pore size was large enough to allow entry of host leukocytes. Furthermore, it was shown that if "immune" lymphoid cells were placed together with target cells in cell-impermeable chambers, which were then inserted into the body cavities of mice having the same genetic constitution as the target tissue grafts, the latter underwent extensive destruction. This was apparently a consequence of an intimate contact between the lymphocytes and the target cells, which led to the destruction of *both.* Subsequent experiments with cell-impermeable diffusion chambers have shown that certain types of ascites tumor cells are destroyed, or their growth is inhibited, when chambers containing them are inserted into hyperimmune hosts. Nevertheless, taken together, these various findings indicate that humoral antibodies probably do not play an important role in solid tissue homograft destruction when present in the concentrations produced after a single exposure to a homograft. Thus skin homografts can be enabled to survive on mice under the protection of treatment with rabbit anti-mouse lymphocyte serum (Chapter 13) despite the fact that such hosts produce fairly high titers of specific H-2 antibodies.

In summary, it appears that, while the destruction of solid tissue homografts is primarily mediated by immunologically competent cells, humoral factors may play an ancillary role, the importance of which varies according to the species, the nature of the target tissue, and the genetic disparity between donor and host.

THE PHENOMENON OF IMMUNOLOGICAL ENHANCEMENT

In the case of certain tumors, and to a lesser extent some normal tissues, including skin, it has been shown that the presence of a high titer of serum antibodies, usually through active immunization with homogenates, dessicates, or other nonliving preparations from a donor strain or through passive transfer of immune serum, may actually *weaken* an animal's ability to react against homografts towards which the humoral antibodies are directed. This is the provocative phenomenon of "immunological *enhancement*" (see Fig. 7.1). Although the nonviable tissue preparations fail to elicit an effective cellular response which is the major factor in graft rejection (see Chapter 8), they apparently do provoke a good humoral response, the essential factor in enhancement. It is interesting to note that Syrian hamsters, which fail to produce demonstrable antibodies when exposed to homografts, do not display the phenomenon of enhancement.

There are marked differences in the ease with which enhancement is demonstrable in different hosts, even within the same species. For example, in mice, C3H or BALB/c strain animals display it much more readily than A strain animals, and it is less easily demonstrated in females than in males of the same isogenic strain. The genetic disparity between the donor and host is also crucially important. When strong histoincompatibility prevails, the immune response provoked by the transplant can usually override any prior enhancing treatment. Furthermore, immunologic enhancement is more easily obtained with certain kinds of tumors than with others. The ease of its induction is inversely related to the extent to which the tumor is sensitive to the cytotoxic action of isoantibody. Thus leukemias are particularly difficult to enhance whereas targets such as most sarcomas, which are less vulnerable to the destructive effects of isoantibody, are easily enhanced.

In most instances what appear to be minor variations in treatment can be crucially important in determining whether an animal becomes enhanced or sensitized. Moreover, animals which manifest an immune response can, with further treatment, sometimes be rendered unresponsive. This suggests that there is a very subtle difference between these two states. For example, mice which have rejected a primary tumor homograft may display an accelerated rate of rejection if reinoculated with the same tumor five to fourteen days later. However, if the interval between the first and second challenge is increased, enhancement of the second graft may occur.

The few direct attempts to prolong the survival of normal solid tissue homografts by enhancement procedures have not been very rewarding. This may be attributed to the fact that skin has usually been the tissue of

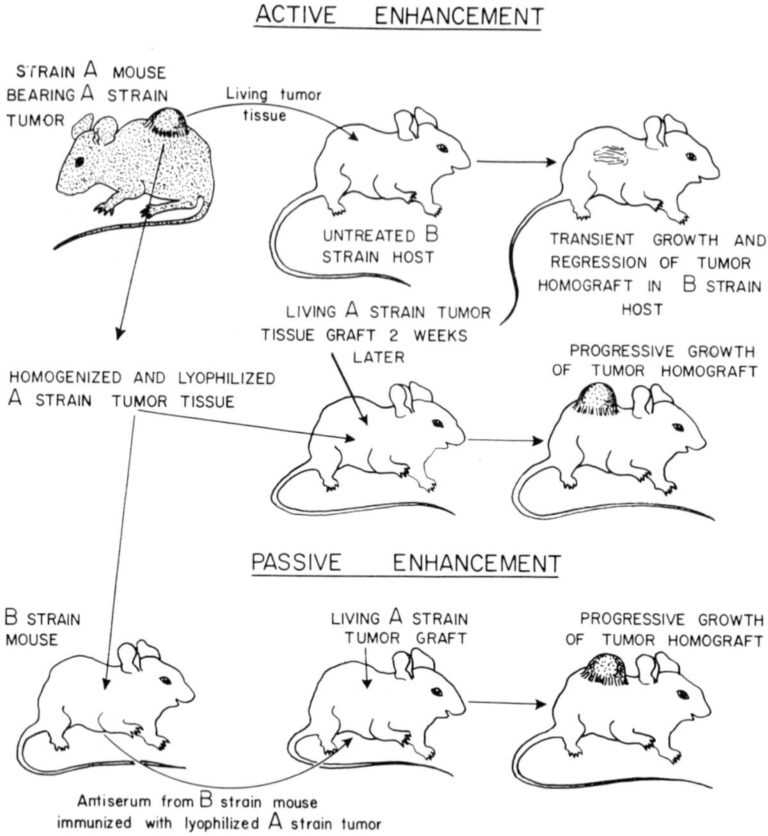

Fig. 7.1. The principal methods of inducing immunological enhancement. In active enhancement, a tumor of A strain origin is removed, homogenized, and freeze-dried (lyophilized). The material is reconstituted in distilled water and inoculated into a B strain host. If untreated, the host would normally reject a challenge graft of A strain tumor tissue. However, as a result of the pretreatment, the B strain mouse sustains the growth of the tumor homograft inoculated two weeks later. In passive enhancement, the lyophilized strain A tumor tissue is first inoculated into a B strain host. This animal is bled two weeks later and its antiserum injected into a second strain B host, which will now accept a homograft of the A strain tumor.

choice in such studies. Probably the best example of enhancement as related to the prolonged survival of skin homografts is that provided by Billingham and Sparrow who found that in adult rabbits the survival of these homografts was increased by a factor of two or three in animals previously inoculated intravenously, but *not* by other routes, with donor epidermal cells or leukocytes in relatively low dosages.

Much more dramatic results have recently been obtained with the enhancement of kidney homografts in rats. For example, Stuart and his associates at the University of Chicago have maintained (Lewis × BN) F_1 hybrid kidneys in Ag-B incompatible, bilaterally nephrectomized, Lewis rats for more than two hundred days by giving them a combined treatment of (1) intravenous injection of donor spleen cells one day before the graft and (2) passive immunization with antiserum prepared in animals of the recipient strain against donor spleen and lymph node cells. French and Batchelor of the McIndoe Memorial Research Unit in East Grinstead, England, have also reported success in enhancing the survival of kidney transplants in Ag-B incompatible rat hosts. They found that 11/11 AS strain rats transplanted with (August × AS) F_1 hybrid kidneys survived for more than 120 days with functioning grafts if they had been inoculated with 1 ml of AS anti-August serum immediately after the operation, 1 ml intraperitoneally 24 hours later, and 0.5 ml, also intraperitoneally, at 48, 72, and 96 hours post-grafting. What is also interesting is that there was a gene-dosage effect since parental strain (August) kidneys did not do as well as (August × AS) F_1 hybrid organs in AS recipients.

Whether similar degrees of enhancement can be expected if such procedures are carried out in man remains to be determined, especially since human kidneys seem to be much more susceptible to the adverse effects of antiserum than those of rats.* Thus it is possible that if employed clinically the enhancing treatment, i.e., the inoculation of antiserum directed against the kidney homograft, would be so deleterious to the transplant itself that it would be unsuitable as an immunosuppressive measure.

The work of Kaliss and his colleagues leaves no doubt whatever that specific antibodies play a fundamental role in the induction of enhancement. There are basically three schools of thought concerning the mode of action of these antibodies: (1) those who believe that the antigenic material released from the graft is prevented from adequately sensitizing the host by virtue of prior union with and preemption by antibodies (afferent inhibition); (2) those who contend that the tumor's antigens reach the reactive lymphoid centers of the host but, as a result of high titers of serum antibodies or of antigen-antibody complexes, these centers are rendered incapable of undertaking a cellular response (central inhibition); and (3) those who believe that the presence of antibodies does not interfere with the development of a cellular response, but that it produces some

* The recent successful prophylactic treatment of Rh negative women who have just given birth to their first Rh positive baby to prevent them from reacting immunologically against subsequent Rh positive fetuses also employs the principle of immunological enhancement. Soon after parturition the women are injected with a small volume of Rh antibody (anti-D) directed against the fetal red cells that have usually gained access to their circulation and would normally sensitize them with respect to subsequent Rh incompatible fetuses.

physiological alteration of the tumor itself so that it is able to evade such a response, e.g., by coating and masking the antigenic determinants on the cells (efferent inhibition).

Evidence that some kind of afferent inhibition is responsible for enhancement stems principally from the observation that the enhanced growth of tumors does not occur if, prior to implantation, the tumor cells are mixed with isologous normal lymph node cells. This suggests that antibodies are unable to wall off the highly mobile lymphocytes in the same manner that they presumably neutralize tumor cells. On the other hand, this hypothesis is difficult to reconcile with the fact that tumors can still be enhanced by antiserum given as late as seven days after the tumor graft, i.e., after antigenic stimulation of the host has presumably occurred. Also in conflict with the afferent hypothesis is the observation that the in vitro exposure of extracted antigens to antiserum does not weaken their power to sensitize in vivo.

Support for the central inhibition and for the afferent inhibition hypothesis stems primarily from an ingenious series of experiments conducted by Snell and his associates, based on an assay developed by Winn. In this assay, presumptively immune lymph node cells, in various dilutions, are mixed with tumor cells and injected into appropriate mice. Immunity is indicated by inhibition of tumor growth. It was found that antiserum given concomitantly with an immunizing tumor homograft depressed the immunity of the cells expressed from the draining nodes to the extent that, at six days after grafting, it was only $\frac{1}{24}$th to $\frac{1}{32}$nd that of cells from controls receiving tumor alone. It seems reasonable, therefore, to assume that this same isoantiserum-mediated depression of cellular immunity is responsible for the continued growth of tumors in enhanced animals. Unfortunately, the same reservations which apply to the afferent inhibition theory apply to the central inhibition hypothesis as well. For example, if some kind of central inhibition is responsible for producing enhancement, it is surprising that antiserum is still able to enhance the growth of tumors as late as seven to ten days after tumor implantation.

The final hypothesis, that of efferent inhibition, received support from observations that: (1) some enhanced tumors display an improved growth, albeit limited in extent, when retransplanted to mice belonging to the tumor's own strain or to animals isogenic with the enhanced hosts but which had previously been actively sensitized with living tumor; (2) enhanced tumors frequently exhibit some loss of strain specificity when retransplanted to normal mice of various strains; and (3) antiserum and immune lymphocytes can be shown to act antagonistically, indicating that antibodies which are not greatly cytotoxic in low concentrations may combine locally with graft antigens and thus disguise the graft cells, protecting them from infiltrating immunologically active host lymphocytes. The major drawback of the efferent inhibition hypothesis is that much of the evidence adduced to support it needs qualifications. For example, some tumors remain unaltered when passaged through enhanced recipients. Furthermore, the change that occurs in other tumors could simply be due to the removal of donor "passenger" leukocytes and other cells from the tumor while it is residing in its enhanced primary host. Lymphocytes are known to be particularly rich in isoantigens, consequently, their absence could reduce the effective immunogenicity of the tumor when it is retransplanted (see Chapter 8).

It is obvious that none of the foregoing hypotheses has as yet achieved decisive predominance over its rivals; each has some measure of experimental support and some serious weaknesses. Only further investigations can reveal the actual mechanism responsible for immunological enhancement.

REFERENCES

Brent, L. 1961. The phenomenon of immunological enhancement, with special reference to immunological tolerance. Estratto da Il Cancro, Periodico dell'Instituto di Oncologia di Torino, 14:1–23.

Hutchin, P. 1968. Mechanisms and functions of immunologic enhancement. Surg. Gynecol., and Obstet. 126:1331–1356.

Kaliss, N. 1958. Immunological enhancement of tumor homografts in mice, a review. Canc. Res. 18:992–1003.

Snell, G. D. 1970. Immunological enhancement. Surg. Gynecol. and Obstet. 130:1109–1119.

Stetson, C. A. 1963. The role of humoral antibody in the homograft reaction. Advances in immunology 3:97–130.

Winn, H. J. 1970. Humoral antibody in allograft reactions. Transpl. Proc. 2:83–91.

Chapter 8

The Mediators of Transplantation Immunity: II. The Role of Lymphocytes

All forms of host reactivity that lead to the destruction of solid tissue homografts, normal or malignant, are almost invariably associated with an infiltration of the alien graft by mononuclear cells of the lymphocytic series and histiocytes. As long ago as 1910, Da Fano realized that this lymphoid reaction had something to do with resistance to grafts. In a classic monograph published in 1926, Dr. James B. Murphy, of the Rockefeller Institute, presented the results of extensive studies on the responses of embryonic and infant chicks, adult mice, and other animals to homografts and heterografts of malignant and normal tissues transplanted to various sites. He concurred with Da Fano that host resistance was evidenced by a round cell reaction about and within the graft, and he noted the absence of this histological hallmark in animals susceptible to the growth of particular tumor grafts. Murphy also investigated the influence of pretreating mice with defibrinated blood, depleting their lymphoid tissue by irradiation, or stimulating it nonspecifically with various agents, on their reactivity to foreign grafts of various types. The results convinced him that ". . . the round cell infiltration so characteristic of the reaction to foreign tissue grafts is a purposeful reaction and that these cells are the agent through which the mechanism exerts its force." Because of his inability to obtain any evidence bearing upon the important question ". . . what the mechanism is that determines whether or not a local reaction is to take place about a cancer graft and how the lymphocyte exerts its influence . . . ," he reluctantly conceded that this cellular reaction might be an associated phenomenon and "not the primary resisting force." Unable to demonstrate the formation of antibodies in any of his experiments, Murphy failed to realize that he was dealing with an immunological phenomenon and used the noncommittal term "resistance."

TRANSFER OF TRANSPLANTATION IMMUNITY

The first piece of solid evidence in support of the thesis that host resistance, or *sensitivity,* to homografts is cell-mediated, as Murphy believed, was produced by Mitchison in 1954. He demonstrated that, whereas a state of actively acquired immunity to tumor homografts in mice was not transferable passively by means of putatively immune serum, even in large amounts, it was transferable "adoptively" by means of *living* (but not killed) cells obtained from mice that had rejected grafts of the tumor. It need hardly be mentioned that for successful transfer of the sensitivity both the donor and the recipient of the cellular "vehicles" *must* be histocompatible. The term "adoptive" immunization was introduced to designate the process whereby a normal subject becomes immune as a result of the transference, not of preformed antibody (i.e., *passive* immunization), but of immunologically activated tissue. It depends upon the presence and *continued* functioning of tissues which had been exposed to an antigenic stimulus in the donor from which they were derived.

These important findings on the transferability of immunity to tumor homografts, soon extended to include homografts of skin (see Fig. 8.1), overcame a serious impasse to progress in our understanding of the homograft reaction by opening up the efferent limb of the immunological reflex to experimental study. They also demonstrated that the *local* or regional lymph nodes are the principal seats of response, or effector organs, against homografts that establish lymphatic connections with their hosts (Fig. 8.2). Equally important was the strength these observations gave to the view, which had slowly been gaining ground on the basis of various lines of indirect evidence, that the homograft reaction, drug and bacterial allergies, states of sensitivity provoked by antigen-antibody complexes, and certain experimental autoimmune reactions, are congeneric phenomena. All of these appear to be characterized by a dual immunological response, one mediated by blood-borne cells, which are responsible for the lesions that characterize them, and the other by the production of humoral antibodies.

In investigations on the adoptive transfer of transplantation immunity, Billingham and his associates found that immunologically tolerant mice and rats (see Chapter 10) could be coerced to reject hitherto healthy, long accepted skin homografts by the transfer of relatively low dosages of regional lymph node cells from either normal or specifically sensitized isologous animals (see Fig. 8.1)—dosages that were very much lower than required to transfer the capacity to give a second-set reaction to a *normal* animal. Cells from sensitized animals abolished tolerance more rapidly than

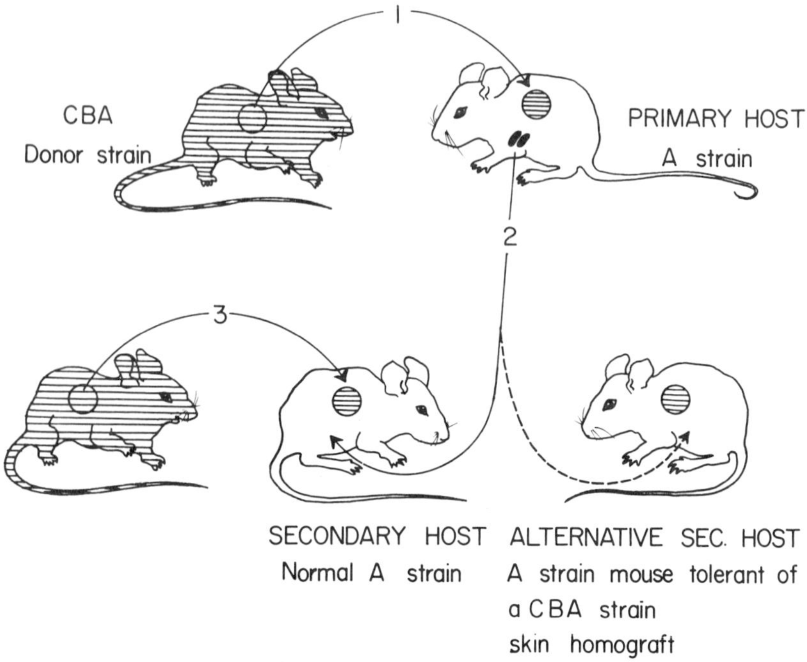

Fig. 8.1. Illustration of the adoptive transfer of transplantation immunity by means of cells from activated regional lymph nodes. (1) A normal A strain mouse is immunized by means of a skin homograft from a CBA donor. (2) Its regional (axillary and brachial) lymph nodes are then excised. A cell suspension is prepared therefrom and injected intraperitoneally into either a normal A mouse, which is challenged with a test graft of CBA skin (3), or an A mouse which has previously been rendered specifically tolerant of a CBA skin graft. Accelerated rejection of its graft by the secondary host, or the prompt rejection of the long-established graft on the alternative secondary (tolerant) host, are indicative of the successful transfer of immunity.

did cells from normal animals, and with appropriate strain combinations, when relatively small numbers of lymphoid cells were transferred, only those from sensitized animals were effective in abolishing tolerance. With the aid of this sensitive experimental system it was shown that whole blood, or leucocyte concentrates prepared therefrom, was as effective as node cells in transferring sensitivity. By means of this system it was also possible to gain some idea of the time of appearance and persistence of "immunologically activated" cells in animals that had received skin homografts. These cells were first demonstrable in the regional nodes and blood of A strain mice, which had received CBA skin grafts, at about the same time—on the sixth day after exposure to the skin homografts. This suggested that the

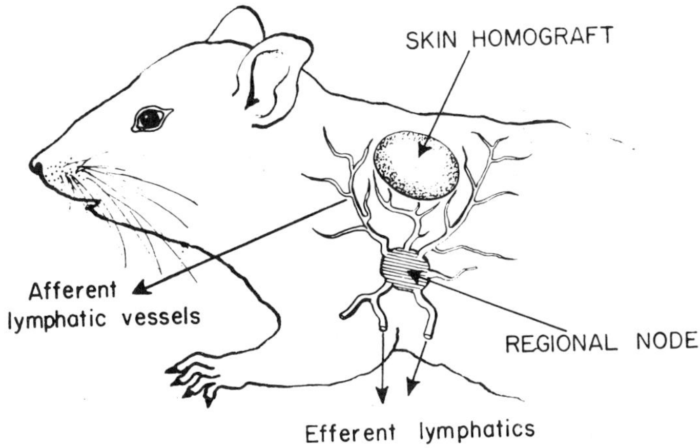

Fig. 8.2. This shows a rat bearing a skin homograft on its thorax and the regional node with its afferent and efferent lymphatic vessels. Presence of the alien graft in its drainage field causes hypertrophy of the node due to either its percolation by antigenic material of graft origin, or the settling in its parenchyma of antigen-reactive lymphocytes, which have been stimulated by antigens in the graft.

cells leave the regional nodes very soon after their formation and enter the circulation. Moreover these activated cells, or postulated *effector cells,* were demonstrable in the host's blood a day or two *before* the development of lesions in the immunizing skin homograft and were still present in both the nodes and the blood as long as a year after graft rejection. The finding that thoracic duct cells (almost exclusively lymphocytes, predominantly of the "small" variety) transferred sensitivity to tolerant rats suggested that the effective cell in the thoracic duct lymph, and in the bloodstream into which it discharges, is a small lymphocyte.

J. L. Gowans found that, in rats, the vast population of small lymphocytes (about 1.5 to 2.0 $\times$ 10^9) which enter the blood stream daily from the thoracic duct are long-lived cells which are constantly recirculating from blood to lymph via the post-capillary venules in the lymph nodes (see Fig. 8.3). In the light of this evidence, it seemed reasonable to conclude that persistent, recirculating, "activated" small lymphocytes were responsible for the long duration of the sensitivity elicited by skin homografts. These biological properties of small lymphocytes also strengthened the view that the second-set reaction expresses a preexisting state of sensitivity rather than a reawakened one. Nevertheless, recognizing that, unlike the immunity evoked by tiny skin homografts transplanted orthotopically, sensitivity induced by small numbers of splenic cells injected intraperi-

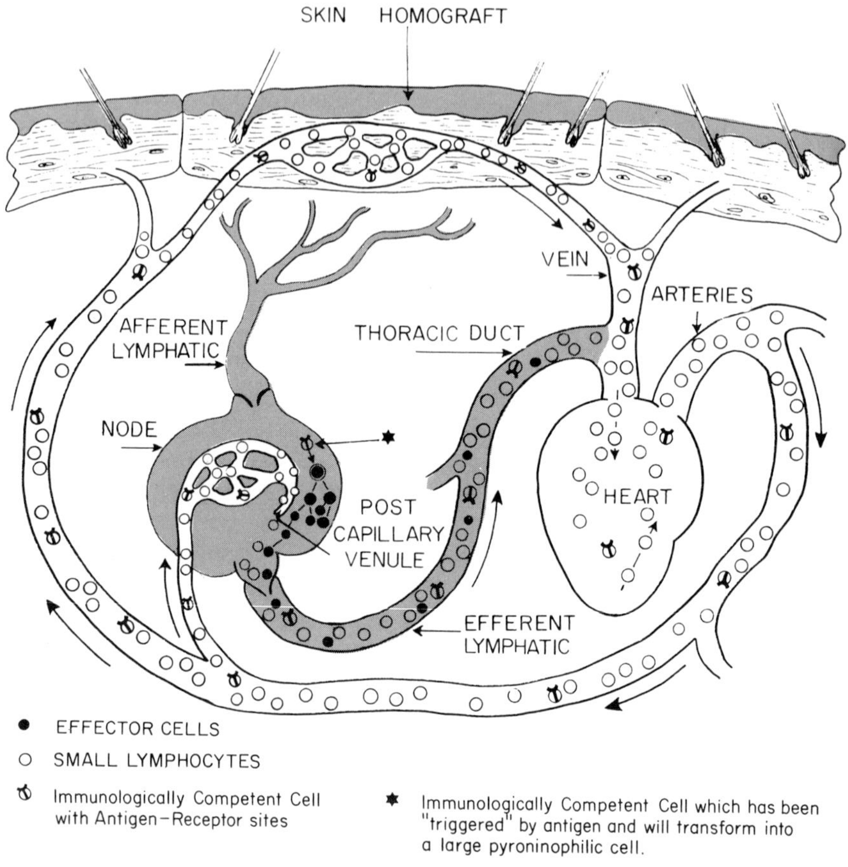

Fig. 8.3. (a) The recirculatory activity of long-lived, small lymphocytes from the blood stream to the lymph via the post-capillary venules in the lymph nodes. (b) Sensitization to a skin homograft. Alien antigenic material from the homograft interacts with specific receptors or recognition units present on the surfaces of some of the small lymphocytes (designated as immunologically competent cells with antigen-receptor sites). After being triggered by antigen, these cells settle out in the regional lymph node and transform into large pyroninophilic cells, or immunoblasts. The latter divide rapidly to form a crop of effector cells (which also have the morphologic characteristics of small lymphocytes). These leave the node via the efferent lymphatics and enter the bloodstream whence they can infiltrate the graft and fulfill their postulated cytopathogenic role.

toneally is dissipated fairly rapidly, Steinmuller was able to show that there is also an anamnestic response in transplantation immunology. In animals sensitized by skin grafts, however, this response probably does not begin to become effective until *after* the demise of a second-set skin graft is almost complete.

Delayed Cutaneous Inflammatory Reactions as Manifestations of Transplantation Immunity

Final and decisive evidence that transplantation immunity is a form of delayed hypersensitivity or allergy came from work initiated by Brent, Brown, and Medawar in 1958. They demonstrated that guinea pigs sensitized by skin homografts respond to subsequent intradermal challenge with living donor cells from the homografts, or antigenic extracts prepared therefrom, with a local dermal inflammatory response of delayed origin—the *direct hypersensitivity reaction* which, both macroscopically and histologically, resembles the classic tuberculin reaction (see Fig. 8.4). Hamsters,

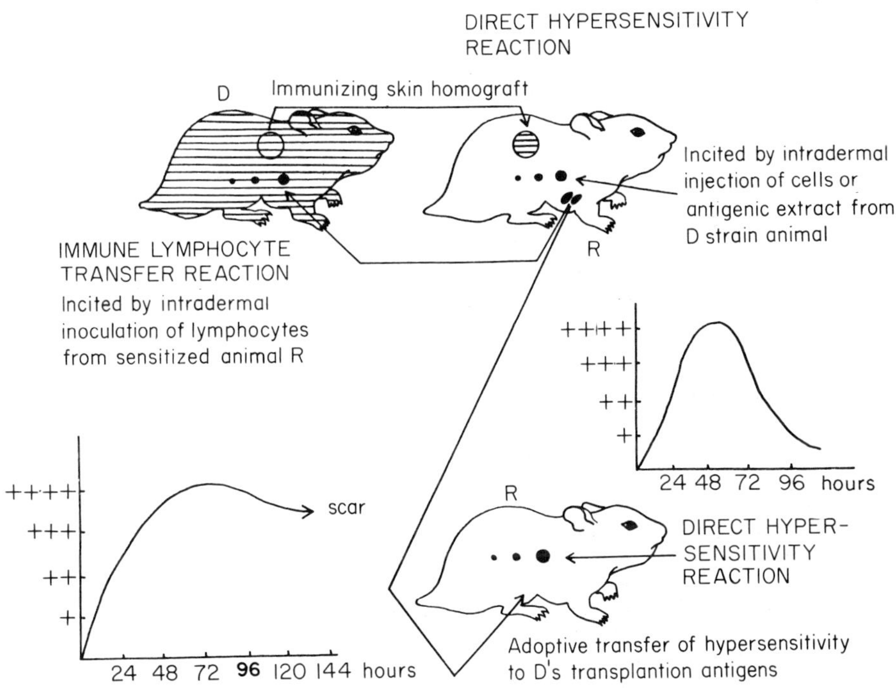

Fig. 8.4. (a) The direct hypersensitivity reaction is incited when viable cells, or subcellular antigenic material, from a donor of strain D are injected intradermally into a hamster of strain R, which has previously been immunized against D strain tissue antigens by means of a skin homograft. Like sensitivity to homografts, the capacity to give a direct reaction is transferable adoptively by means of viable lymphoid tissue cells but not by means of putatively immune serum. (b) An immune lymphocyte transfer reaction is incited if a suspension of lymphoid cells from a specifically sensitized hamster, R, is injected into the skin of the animal against whose tissue antigens its immunity is directed. The time courses of typical direct hypersensitivity reactions and immune lymphocyte transfer reactions are shown in the right and left graphs, respectively.

mice, rats, cattle, and other species behave similarly though there are wide variations in the intensity of the erythematous component of these reactions. It was also discovered that, if a suspension of lymphoid cells—preferably lymphocytes from the peripheral blood—from animals specifically sensitized by means of skin grafts are injected intradermally into the graft *donor,* essentially similar reactions ensue. These are known as *immune lymphocyte transfer* (ILT) *reactions* (Fig. 8.4) and are interpreted as the result of a *local* interaction between the transferred immunologically activated cells and the transplantation antigens of the donor. ILT reactions, which are local *graft-versus-host* (GVH) *reactions* (see Chapter 11), cannot be incited by serum or by devitalized lymphocytes from sensitized donors.

Both the direct reaction and the ILT reaction have latent periods of about five to eight hours and attain their peak intensities within twenty-four to forty-eight hours. They are highly specific immunologically and their intensities reflect the strengths of the homograft reactions responsible for their evocation. The magnitude and time course of ILT reactions are determined by the number of cells transferred, and the reactions frequently culminate in the partial or complete necrosis of the lesions produced.

In guinea pigs, hamsters, and certain other species including man, lymphocytes from *normal* adult donors injected intradermally into normal homologous hosts may also incite inflammatory reactions of delayed origin known as *normal lymphocyte transfer* (NLT) *reactions* (Fig. 8.5). These reactions (also discussed in Chapters 2 and 11), which may be discernible as early as fifteen hours after inoculation, are also GVH reactions as indicated, for example, by their development when lymphocytes of parental strain origin are injected into the skins of F_1 hybrid hosts.

Contrary to expectation, various lines of evidence have indicated that the native or indigenous cell population in the host's skin makes no significant contribution to either ILT or NLT reactions. Hamsters made highly leukopenic by irradiation fail to give these reactions. However, if a usually effective number of normal or sensitized donor lymphocytes are mixed with viable cells or antigenic extracts of the host's genetic constitution and are then injected into heavily irradiated animals, NLT and ILT reactions, respectively, develop. This suggests that in unirradiated hosts immigrant cells of hematogenous origin enter the inoculation sites and furnish the antigenic stimulus.

On the basis of extensive comparative studies on the ILT and NLT reactions in guinea pigs, too extensive to summarize here, Medawar and Brent have formulated an ingenious quantal theory of the action of lymphocytes. They suggest that immunologically competent small lymphocytes and the population of sensitized lymphocytes to which they give rise by proliferation following antigenic stimulation (see Fig. 8.3) are qualitatively

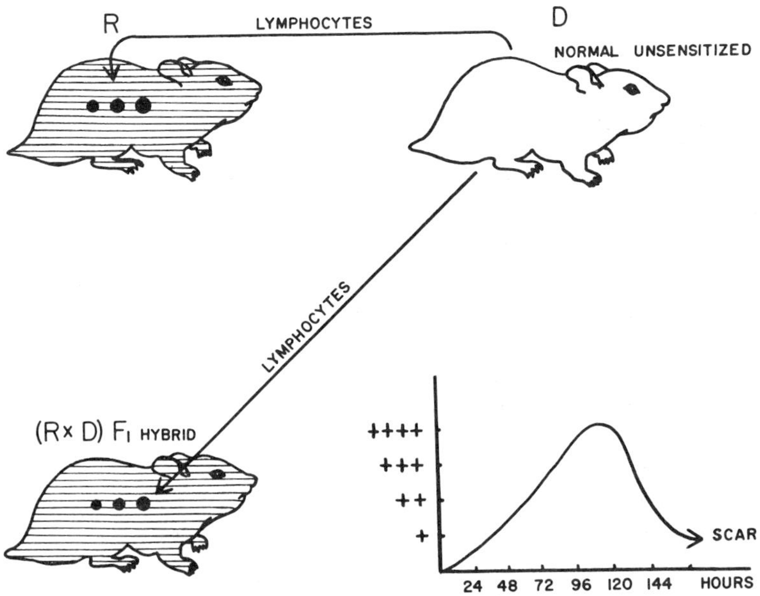

Fig. 8.5. Normal lymphocyte transfer reactions are incited when lymphocytes from a normal unsensitized hamster, D, are injected into the skin of an unrelated hamster of strain R, or of an (R × D) F_1 hybrid. Use of the genetically tolerant hybrid host ensures that the cutaneous reactions which develop at the inoculation sites are exclusively those caused by the response of D's immunologically competent cells against alien transplantation antigens which the hybrid has inherited from its R strain parent. The graph illustrates the development of the intensity of the cutaneous inflammatory reaction with time after inoculation.

similar. The only difference between a sensitized and a normal animal, according to their reasoning, is that the former contains a much higher proportion of lymphocytes that can react with a particular antigen. The early inflammatory component of the NLT reaction is interpreted as a manifestation of an immunological "recognition" event on the part of those immunologically competent cells present which were innately endowed with the capacity to recognize and interact with the antigens of the particular host concerned. Activation of these cells leads to their proliferation to produce a significant population of like cells whose activity is responsible for intensification of the overt NLT reaction which commences after about the fourth day.

Their findings also suggest that, irrespective of whether the sensitivity of a host is directed against strong or weak transplantation antigens, on a cell-for-cell basis, *sensitized* lymphocytes are equivalent with respect to their capacity to harm target cells or organs. This interesting concept is consonant with Simonsen's thesis that the strength of a histocompatibility antigen is a reflection of the number (or proportion) of cells in the unsensitized animal initially capable of recognizing and reacting with it.

Until fairly recently it was believed that the distribution of immunologically competent cells was restricted to the various lymphoid tissues of the body and the bone marrow. However, using the capacity of cells to cause GVH reactions as a criterion (see Chapter 11), it was found that normal peripheral blood contains immunologically competent, or antigen-sensitive, cells having the morphological characteristics of small lymphocytes. Various observations indicate that these cells are part of the recirculating pool of long-lived small lymphocytes which, though thymus-derived, are ultimately of bone marrow origin (see Chapter 9).

Procedures that deplete an animal's pool of recirculating lymphocytes, which include whole-body irradiation, extracorporeal irradiation of its blood or lymph, chronic thoracic duct drainage, neonatal thymectomy, thymectomy in adult life followed by whole-body irradiation, or treatment with antilymphocyte serum (see Chapter 13) weaken its capacity to reject homografts, or the capacity of its lymphoid tissue cells to incite GVH reactions. Restoration of competence to react against homografts can be achieved by transfusion of thoracic duct cells.

Various lines of evidence, some of which are described below, indicate that, when antigen-sensitive small lymphocytes are confronted by alien transplantation antigens, some kind of specific "recognition" process occurs, probably mediated by preformed antibody-like receptor units, sometimes referred to as immunoglobulin X, on their surfaces (see Fig. 8.3). As a result, a small proportion are triggered or activated, their peregrination from blood to lymph ceases, and they take up residence in lymphoid tissues—predominantly in the regional nodes when skin and subcutaneously implanted homografts are concerned. Here the activated cells promptly transform into large pyroninophilic cells, or *immunoblasts,* which, by brisk mitotic activity, give rise to a population of lymphocytes of progressively smaller size. These enter the bloodstream via the efferent lymphatics, thus joining the recirculating lymphocyte pool (see Chapter 9) whence they are free to traverse the vasculature of the alien graft responsible for their genesis and fulfill their role as specific effector cells.

Not unreasonably, following the demonstration of the transferability of sensitivity to homografts by means of regional lymph node cells, or blood-borne cells, it became generally assumed that the infiltrating mononuclear cell population in a homograft reflects the gathering of an immunologically specific population of effector cells, generated predominantly in the regional nodes, which have "homed" specifically into the alien target graft.

Alas, this simple picture has been shown to be a complete misrepresentation. The application of radioisotope techniques to study the infiltrating cell population in primary skin homografts confirmed that the small lymphocytes present are mainly *new* cells, many of which are formed in the regional nodes in response to the graft. However, as Dr. Robert Prendergast demonstrated so clearly, the apparent predilection of the vast majority of these newly formed cells for homografts is not immunologically specific. Thus if the regional auricular lymph node draining a skin homograft on one ear of a rabbit is carefully labeled by injection of tritiated thymidine into the graft, small lymphocytes formed in this node will just as readily enter a skin homograft from another, *unrelated,* donor concomitantly transplanted to the contralateral ear. Moreover, labeled lymphocytes, formed in the node stimulated by the skin homograft, will enter with equal facility the site of a delayed hypersensitivity reaction against a heterologous protein antigen with respect to which the host had previously been sensitized. Up to 11% of the mononuclear cells infiltrating the homografts and the site of the delayed hypersensitivity reaction were labeled, whereas only a small proportion of mononuclear cells in the blood were labeled.

Consistent with these important findings, and making the cellular response to homografts even more difficult to interpret, is the evidence that, when sensitivity to skin homografts is transferred adoptively by means of tagged cells to normal hosts, or to specifically tolerant animals bearing foreign grafts, exceedingly few labeled cells are demonstrable among the cells which infiltrate the target skin homografts. There are two possible interpretations of this situation: either (1) the sensitized cells, when injected systemically, may have properties that oblige them to become localized in lymphoid tissue, and it is their unlabeled *descendants* that attack the graft, or (2) the vast majority of the cells, which have infiltrated a graft undergoing destruction due to adoptive immunization of its host, comprises immunologically uncommitted host cells, probably including a large proportion of cells of bone marrow origin. This latter possibility implies that infiltration of a homograft by a very small number of "committed" cells suffices to procure its destruction. It leaves us, however, with the problem of explaining the possible role of the abundant, apparently uncommitted cells which, depending upon the experimental design, may be immunologically incompetent. A similar state of affairs occurs in delayed hypersensitivity reactions.

Several lines of evidence suggest that these "uncommitted" cells are in some way essential and play an important role in the lesions which develop at antigen test sites in the direct reaction and in other delayed hypersensitivity reactions. For example, dosages of lymph node cells from specifically sensitized animals, which would normally transfer the capacity to give *direct reactions* to normal isologous hosts, are ineffective if the latter have been heavily irradiated.

The Site of Antigen Recognition

Apart from the nature of the antigen-recognition process about which little is known, another important question relates to the site where this important confrontation between antigen-sensitive cells and graft antigen actually takes place. So far as skin grafts are concerned, the conventional belief was that sensitization is elicited by percolation of antigenic material, traveling from the grafts via peripheral lymphatics, through the nodes (see Figs. 8.2 and 8.3). However, on the basis of the evidence that immunologically competent cells are normal ingredients of blood, Medawar suggested that sensitization may take place *peripherally,* possibly at the level of the graft's vascular endothelium. Lymphocytes activated within the graft may then traverse its parenchyma and reach the nodes via lymphatic pathways, where they settle and generate the effector cell population.

So far as orthotopic homografts of skin are concerned, the presence of an intact lymphatic drainage in the graft bed seems essential for sensitization to occur. Evidence sustaining this statement is the anomalous survival of vascularized skin homografts in hamsters' cheek pouches and in the skin flaps prepared in the flank skin of guinea pigs (see Chapter 5); these are sites which lack lymphatic drainage.

What has to pass down the lymphatics to cause sensitization of the host remains to be established. Is it antigenic material or peripherally activated lymphocytes? Hall has shown that in sheep the lymph draining the sites of fresh grafts of homologous skin toward the regional nodes contains large amounts of cell debris but relatively few leucocytes (1000/mm^3, 75% of which are macrophages).

In the case of *organ* homografts which are immediately revascularized by surgical anastomoses, an intact lymphatic drainage system does not seem to be required for sensitization. In dogs both heart and renal homografts, invested in plastic bags in such a way as to preclude the regeneration of lymphatic channels, are rejected in a normal manner. Furthermore, Drs. Ballantyne and Nathan have shown that exposure of rats to ex vivo renal homografts for as little as thirty minutes can provoke detectable levels of sensitivity, and in man the rejection of an extracorporeal kidney connected to the host by silastic tubing has been observed.

Although such findings as these indicate that renal homografts provide their immunogenic influence via the venous route, they afford no clue as to the identity of the agent(s) involved. On the basis of tests carried out on the plasma and cellular fractions of the venous effluent of canine renal homografts for their ability to sensitize other dogs, Dr. John Najarian and his associates have suggested that antigenic material might be in the plasma component.

What has been widely accepted as strong evidence for the concept of peripheral sensitization was presented by Drs. Strober and Gowans. They perfused either whole blood or lymphoid cells of rats of one strain through isolated kidneys derived from rats of another inbred strain, returning the blood or cells to rats of the original donor strain. When subsequently challenged with skin homografts of the same origin as the perfused kidneys, these animals gave evidence of sensitivity. Although Strober and Gowans took pains to flush out residual blood cells from the donor kidneys *before* in vitro perfusion, the possibility remains that the sensitivity they observed was in response to residual passenger leucocytes carried into the host via the blood or lymphocyte suspension. It is pertinent to mention here that even after perfusion of 2 ml of saline through a freshly excised rat kidney, as many as 0.5×10^6 leucocytes can subsequently be washed out with further perfusion.

The Role of Passenger Cells in Sensitization

The possibility that donor leucocytes, probably of the mononuclear series, inadvertently transferred in the vasculature and probably to some extent in the extravascular spaces of tissue and organ grafts, may provide a significant antigenic stimulus to a recipient is now under active consideration. Evidence that cells of hematogenous origin, rather than *native* cells in the host's skin, are the incitants of both NLT and ILT reactions in hamsters pointed in this direction. More cogent, perhaps, was the finding by Elkins and Guttman that Lewis parental strain lymphocytes deposited beneath the renal capsules of orthotopically transplanted Lewis kidneys in genetically tolerant (BN $\times$ Lewis) F_1 hosts caused local destructive lesions. In this situation the attacking cells and the renal parenchyma into which they were deposited were of the *same* antigenic constitution (see Chapter 11); hence, the only possible source of the antigenic stimulus was the circulating leucocytes of the F_1 hybrid host. Moreover, as Guttman and his colleagues have shown, rejection is delayed when Lewis rats receive genetically incompatible (BN $\times$ Lewis) F_1 kidneys from animals which have had their marrow replaced by cells of Lewis origin.

Dr. David Steinmuller has recently demonstrated that the relatively small population of passenger donor leucocytes harbored in the vasculature of free skin grafts in mice is sufficient to incite sensitivity. Using animals that were chimeric with respect to their lymphohematopoietic tissues and blood leukocytes as donors, he found that transfer of skin from them to normal animals of their own strain resulted in sensitization of the latter to tissue antigens of the strain which donated the cells responsible for producing the chimerism initially (see Fig. 8.6). He also found that the sensi-

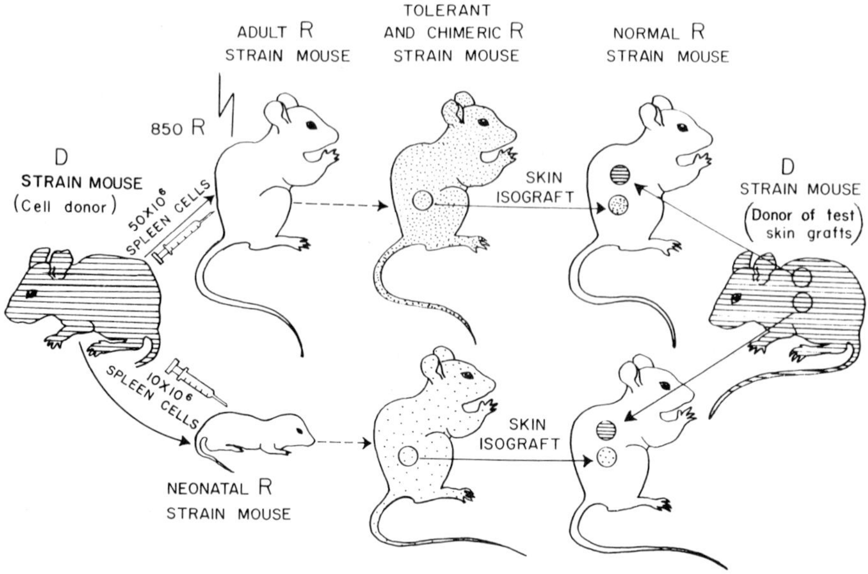

Fig. 8.6. The experimental design used by Dr. David Steinmuller to demonstrate the immunogenicity of passenger cells in skin grafts. R strain mice are rendered chimeric with respect to lymphohematopoietic cells from D strain donors, either by lethal X-irradiation, followed by a transfusion of D strain marrow cells (top row of mice) or by neonatal injection with D strain splenic cells (bottom row of mice). If skin isografts are subsequently transferred from chimeric R strain mice to normal R strain mice, the latter are found to reject subsequent test skin homografts from a D strain donor in an accelerated manner. This is indicative of the transfer of "contaminating" D strain leucocytes in the skin grafts from the chimeric R strain donors.

tizing capacity of the skin isografts was greatly diminished if they were removed from chimeric mice previously made leukopenic by irradiation.

Various lines of evidence indicate that, so far as *skin* homografts are concerned, passenger cells play at most only a minor role in host sensitization. For example, sheets of pure epidermis, isolated enzymically from the dermis and grafts of cornea (a specialized type of skin), both of which are totally devoid of blood vessels and, therefore, of significant numbers of contaminating passenger cells, are rejected in a normal manner if transplanted to recipient areas prepared in the integument of homologous hosts.

However, since tissues and organs undoubtedly differ considerably in their immunogenicity and susceptibility to rejection, the role of passenger leucocytes in determining their fate may be more important for some than for others. Firstly, leucocytes may provide a potent *local* antigenic stimulus for peripheral sensitization, which may to some extent result from a tendency of host responding cells to enter into the sort of intimate contactual relationships with them that occur in mixed leucocyte interactions in vitro (see Chapter 2). Second, many of the passenger cells are probably swept along by the host's blood, gaining access to its lymphoid centers where they bring their immunogenicity to bear *centrally*.

In the case of grafts of low intrinsic immunogenicity, such as hearts in Ag-B locus-compatible rats, removal of their passenger cells by experimental artifice may well reduce both their capacity to elicit transplantation immunity as well as their susceptibility to it.

It is worth pointing out that, if peripheral sensitization is a valid phenomenon, it constitutes an effective host recognition mechanism for grafts of long standing in immunosuppressed hosts, after cessation of treatment, provided that (1) appropriate antigen-sensitive cells are present in the host and (2) some kind of graft adaptation (see Chapter 6), possibly as a consequence of the insidious replacement of its vascular endothelial cells by those of the host, has not taken place.

Studies by both light and electron microscopy of homografts undergoing rejection have proved exceedingly unrewarding from the viewpoint of revealing any causal relationship between the mononuclear cell infiltrate and the lesion with which it is so intimately associated. In fact, with few exceptions, the proximate cause of death of a homograft remains open to speculation. Local accumulation of mononuclear cells, both inside and outside vessel walls, and a direct cytopathic action of these cells on the foreign cell population of the graft, whether in the vessel walls, connective tissue, or epidermis, have been cited as contributory factors.

Studies of several local GVH reaction systems, such as the NLT and ILT reactions and others to be described in Chapter 11, have established that sensitization may occur locally and, more important, may lead to *local* tissue lesions of varying severity. This affords fairly convincing evidence of the capacity of lymphocytes to inflict overt damage directly on target tissue in vivo.

Early evidence for the postulated cytopathogenic effect of lymphocytes was furnished more than a decade ago by the late Dr. Glen Algire and his colleagues. This has been described on page 96.

Another important indication of the destructive potentiality of lymphoid cells in vivo was obtained by Dr. Henry Winn. He mixed target homologous tumor cell suspensions with node cells from specifically immunized mice and then inoculated the mixtures into appropriate hosts. Suppression of tumor cell growth was demonstrable with node cell/tumor cell ratios as low as 1:10. Particularly important was his demonstration that the immune node cells were more effective in suppressing tumor cell growth when actually mixed with the target cells than when inoculated separately at different sites, suggesting that contact or at least close association was necessary.

As the evidence mounted that some diffusible agent(s), in some way associated with lymphocytes, was responsible for the destruction of homografts, attempts were made to extract it, first to verify its existence, and second as an essential step in its characterization. In the experience of most investigators the use of *living* sensitized cells to transfer transplantation immunity or incite ILT reactions has been obligatory. Intact but devitalized cells, subcellular homogenates, or extractives have proved ineffective. This might suggest that the agent(s) which is responsible for the homograft reaction is not produced until after the activated lymphocytes have actually been engaged by antigen. The fact that both the NLT and the ILT reactions and the direct reaction are of the "delayed" type hints that the mobilized population of effector cells may require time to synthesize effective amounts of the putative effector.

Two groups of investigators have reported that sensitivity to skin homografts is transferable adoptively in mice, guinea pigs, and rabbits by means of large numbers of isologous sensitized lymphoid cells imprisoned in small, cell-impermeable Millipore chambers inserted subcutaneously or intraperitoneally. However, independent attempts to confirm these potentially important findings have been unsuccessful.

Dr. R. A. Good and his associates have recently reported the successful transfer of transplantation immunity in mice by means of small volumes of plasma from isologous donors which, after sensitization to the tissue antigens of an unrelated strain, are subjected to whole-body irradiation. These workers suggest that the irradiation releases a normally cell-bound antibody-like (thymus-dependent) factor responsible for the cellular immunity into the plasma. Normal, isologous spleen cells incubated in vitro with plasma from sensitized and irradiated animals are capable of absorbing this factor and, even after washing, are themselves capable of transferring sensitivity. These findings, which are similar to previous ones on the transfer of delayed allergy to tuberculin in guinea pigs, do not entirely exclude the possibility that the agent involved is in fact antigenic material released from the donor by irradiation, and that the sensitivity alleged to be of passive origin is in fact actively acquired by the plasma recipients. Consistent with this interpretation is the fact that Lubaroff and Silvers have been unable to abolish tolerance of skin homografts in mice with plasma from irradiated donors which have been specifically sensitized against the antigens of the tolerance-conferring donor.

In Vitro Studies

Convincing evidence that lymphocytes from sensitized animals can destroy target cells from donors against whose antigens the sensitivity is directed has been furnished by numerous in vitro studies following the pioneer work of Govaerts and of Rosenau and Moon in 1960. For example, when suspensions of splenic cells, lymph node cells, peritoneal exudate cells, or thoracic duct cells from immunized animals are added to monolayers of target cells attached to glass, within a matter of hours, lymphocytes begin to cluster around the target cells—a phenomenon known as "contactual agglutination." Subsequently, affected target cells retract their cytoplasmic processes, round up, and become detached from their substrate as a consequence of some kind of cytolytic process. This cytocidal attribute of the attacking lymphocytes is highly specific immunologically, requiring neither added complement nor specific antibody. What seems to be essential is intimate contact between attacking and target cells, and this may be the only component of the cell-to-cell interaction that is immunologically specific. On the basis of carefully designed quantitative experiments, Dr. Darcy Wilson concluded that a single lymphocyte, if immunologically activated, is sufficient to harm one target cell, and that 1 to 2% of the cells present in the regional lymph nodes of a sensitized rat are immunologically active in this sense.

Another useful procedure for revealing transplantation immunity in vitro was developed by Dr. Herman Friedman. It is based on the fact that spleen cell suspensions from mice (of strain A, say), immunized with sheep red blood cells, form localized foci of hemolysis (known as antibody plaques), when incubated in an agar gel containing sheep erythrocytes and complement. If, however, the putative homolysin-producing spleen cells are first incubated with spleen cells from a mouse of strain B, which has been immunized against the tissue antigens of strain A, plaque formation is inhibited due to the expression of homograft reactivity.

Apart from establishing the specific cytopathogenic potentiality of sensitized lymphocytes, in vitro work by numerous investigators has now revealed that when activated lymphocytes from animals made delayed hypersensitive to a variety of antigens, including those responsible for transplantation immunity, are confronted by the antigen concerned, they synthesize and release into the culture medium diffusible, immunologically nonspecific, biologically, or pharmacologically active agents. These have been recognized in terms of their ability to inhibit the migration of macrophages (MIF or macrophage inhibition factor), actually kill cells (lymphotoxins), stimulate lymphocytes to transform preparatory to division (blastogenic factor), exert a chemotactic influence on mononuclear cells, or incite delayed-type inflammatory reactions when injected into the skins of guinea pigs or hamsters.

In addition to these agents which are released when antigen-activated cells are confronted by antigen in tissue culture, extensive studies by Granger and others have shown that lymphocytes from *unsensitized* donors may also release lymphotoxins when cultured with any of an extensive and varied number of agents that induce blastogenic transformation, whether specifically (as in the mixed lymphocyte interaction) or nonspecifically (e.g., by phytohemagglutinin). Following an initial triggering or initiating step, active metabolism and synthesis on the part of the stimulated lymphocyte seem to be involved.

In summary, recent work has now confirmed the long-postulated, contact-dependent cytopathogenic effect of sensitized lymphocytes. It has also established that less intimate degrees of exposure of both normal and sensitized lymphocyte populations to homologous cellular antigens can initiate the synthesis and release of a variety of diffusible, immunologically nonspecific agents capable of affecting the well-being and behavior of neighboring cells, irrespective of their genetic constitution. Some of these agents incite vascular permeability changes and inflammation in vivo.

There is an urgent need for purification, chemical definition, and discriminating tests to determine exactly how many there are of these agents. At present a factor tends to be defined in the particular context in which it is revealed, leaving open the question whether several of the agents so defined are really one and the same substance. Finally, of course, we need to know exactly what role these agents play in homograft reactivity in vivo. One can now begin to see how, following the arrival of a few sensitized lymphocytes in a homograft, and their interaction and engagement with target cells, diffusible mediators may help to recruit, trap, and direct the activities of a considerable heterogeneous population of cells of hematogenous origin leading to death of the graft.

With certain immunological reactions that are antibody-mediated, at least two types of cells are involved. Antigen has to be trapped and processed in some way by macrophages before it can induce the activation of lymphocytes. At present we do not know whether two types of cell are required for the release of the various putative effector molecules considered above. Indeed, there is no critical evidence bearing upon the important question of whether macrophages, which like small lymphocytes are a heterogeneous group of cells of different origins, play any essential role in the process of homograft rejection. Present opinion suggests that in the case of normal tissues and organs they do not, but recent studies, particularly by Weiser's group at Seattle, have implicated immunologically specific activity of macrophages in the rejection of some ascites tumors.

Since, in adoptive transfer experiments, it has been fairly well established that the vast majority of mononuclear cells that invade the target grafts are unsensitized host cells, the question remains whether these cells are merely spectators of the tragedy about to unfold or whether, because of possible "priming" activities on the part of the minority of sensitized cells, they are enlisted as active participants. The mediators we've just considered afford a possible mechanism whereby this could take place.

Other agents are known that might fulfill an instructional role by transmitting immunological "information." For example, Dr. H. S. Lawrence and his colleagues at New York University Medical School have shown that, in man, an agent they've described as "transfer factor" is extractable from peripheral blood leucocytes of persons sensitized to transplantation antigens or other delayed allergens. Transfer factor is a small, nonantigenic, nonimmunoglobulin molecule (molecular weight $< 10,000$) apparently capable of transferring to some portion of the lymphocyte population of an unsensitized individual, either in vivo or in vitro, the specific actively acquired immunological memories of the donor. Sensitivity acquired through transfer factor is long lasting.

The second candidate is RNA. Drs. Mannick and Egdahl first made the interesting observation that, in rabbits, sensitized immunologic status can be conferred upon normal lymph node cells by treatment in vitro with RNA extracted from node cells of rabbits that have rejected skin homografts. Subsequently, Wilson and Wecker demonstrated that, in rats, RNA from "immune" lymphoid cells will convert isologous normal lymphocytes to "immune" status so that they manifest weak though definite cytocidal activity against appropriate target cells in vitro.

McFarland and his group have shown that lymphocytes may establish cytoplasmic bridges with neighboring cells in tissue culture via their so-called foot appendages or "uropods." These bridges may transmit "informational" molecules of the kind under consideration.

Mixed Lymphocyte Interactions

Apart from its value as a histocompatibility matching procedure (see Chapter 2), the mixed leucocyte interaction test has afforded an invaluable approach for analyzing the events that follow the stimulation of antigen-sensitized lymphocytes by cellular transplantation antigens. The most useful experimental situation is that afforded when parental strain lymphocytes are mixed with those from F_1 hybrid donors so that *one-way* reactions take place. Advantage has been taken of chromosomal markers to define the origin of the reacting cells. Critical studies have established that the cells which undergo blastoid transformation and subsequent proliferation are small lymphocytes and that the response is immunologically specific. Lymphocytes from F_1 hybrid animals are incapable of responding against parental strain cells, even in an environment in which other cells are proliferating. Moreover, lymphocytes from tolerant animals are incapable of responding against cells from donors with respect to whose antigens they are unresponsive. However, they do respond against cells from donors of a different, unrelated strain. That the lymphocytes from neonatally thymectomized animals do not respond in mixed cell culture indicates the thymic dependency of the reacting cells.

As already mentioned, an essential prerequisite for significant levels of MLI activity is confrontation of the putative responder cells by antigens determined by the major H-locus for the species concerned. For example, if lymphocytes from two Ag-B compatible rat strains are mixed, the cells fail to respond in vitro.

The total proportion of cells initially present in a culture that are capable of responding to a major H-locus incompatibility has been shown to be of the order of 1 to 3%, though not all of these cells begin to respond at the same time. This figure is comparable with the proportion of peripheral blood lymphocytes from adult chickens capable of GVH reactivity in embryos confronting them with a strong histocompatibility antigen.

The most plausible explanation for the failure of mixed lymphocyte interactions to occur when only nonmajor H-locus incompatibilities prevail is that, in such situations, the proportion of lymphocytes in the circulating pool capable of reacting is too low to be revealed in in vitro systems. The high proportion of lymphocytes capable of responding to antigens determined by major loci may be a function of the multiple specificities associated with the various alleles (see Chapters 1 and 3), though this is clearly not the complete explanation.

So far, no convincing evidence has been forthcoming that the cells which are stimulated to proliferate, or their progeny, are activated lymphocytes or specific effector cells, capable of inflicting damage upon their target cells or of transferring sensitivity adoptively. However, Dr. Haim Ginsburg has recently reported that, under certain conditions, when small lymphocytes from *unsensitized* rats are cultured on monolayers of homologous fibroblasts, a large proportion transform to blastoid cells. The latter subsequently differentiate into large pyroninophilic cells capable of lysing target cells. These pyroninophilic cells could be harvested and transferred to fresh target cell monolayers whose components they were able to lyse within sixteen hours. This represents a complete in vitro model of homograft reactivity since both the initiation and the effectuation of the lymphocytic response take place in vitro.

REFERENCES

Brent, L., and P. B. Medawar. 1967. Cellular immunity and the homograft reaction. Brit. Med. Bull. 23:55–60.

Lawrence, H. S., and M. Landy [ed.]. 1969. Mediators of cellular immunity. Academic Press, New York.

Murphy, J. B. 1926. The lymphocyte in resistance to tissue grafting, malignant disease, and tuberculous infection. Monog. 21. The Rockefeller Institute for Medical Research, New York.

Roitt, I. M., M. F. Greaves, G. Torrigiani, J. Brostoff, and J. H. Playfair. 1969. The cellular basis of immunological responses. Lancet ii:367–371.

Wilson, D. B., and R. E. Billingham. 1967. Lymphocytes and transplantation immunity. Advances in Immunol. 7:189–273.

Chapter 9

The Thymus and Transplantation Immunity

"It has fallen to my lot to show that the first leucocytes arise in the thymus, from its epithelial cells, and that the thymus must be regarded as the parent source of all the lymphoid structures of the body. It does not cease to exist in later life no more than would the Anglo-Saxon race disappear were the British Isles to sink beneath the waves. For just as the Anglo-Saxon stock has made its way from its original home into all parts of the world, and has there set up colonies for itself and for its increase, so the original leucocytes, starting from their birth place in the thymus, have penetrated into almost every part of the body, and have there created new centres for growth, for increase, and useful work for themselves and for the body. . . ."—J. BEARD, 1899.

Although the seat of the soul has long been a bone of contention to philosophers, most transplantation immunologists would agree that at least a major part of it must reside in the thymus gland—a bi-lobed structure that lies in the upper chest in front of the aorta. This is because the principal function of this lymphoid organ, which as recently as ten years ago was unknown, lies in the predominant role it plays in controlling the maturation and maintenance of that part of the lymphoid system which is responsible for *cell*-mediated immunological reactions including, of course, that responsible for homograft reactivity. Thus, though Dr. J. Beard, as long ago as 1899, presented an amazingly accurate picture of the functional significance of the thymus, based on purely histological studies in an elasmobranch, it was not until this decade that his contention that this organ was intimately involved with lymphopoiesis received experimental confirmation.

INFLUENCE OF NEONATAL THYMECTOMY

The initial series of experiments which focused attention on the vital role the thymus plays in the development of immunity were carried out almost simultaneously by J. F. A. P. Miller, who was then working at the

Chester Beatty Research Institute in London, and by the late Carlos Martinez and his colleagues at the University of Minnesota. Miller removed the thymus in one group of C3H and Ak mice within one to sixteen hours after birth and in another group at five days of age.* At six weeks of age both groups of animals, as well as sham-thymectomized and entirely normal mice, were challenged with skin grafts, Ak mice receiving C3H grafts, and vice versa. The MST of skin grafts in the intact and sham-thymectomized mice, and in animals thymectomized at five days of age, ranged from ten to twelve days. On the other hand, in more than 70% of the mice whose thymuses had been removed on the first day of life, the grafts became established and grew luxuriant crops of fur. Most of these grafts were accepted for periods ranging from six weeks to two months and some for even longer periods. Miller also noted that these neonatally thymectomized animals were lymphopenic.

Martinez obtained similar results but, in addition, found that with certain H-2 compatible mouse strain combinations, some animals thymectomized as late as thirty days after birth accepted skin homografts for prolonged periods.

These experiments, which indicated that neonatal thymectomy results in a depletion of lymphocytes and in serious immunological defects in the mature animal, set the stage for a whole battery of investigations, many of which are still in progress, to determine the means by which these effects are mediated. Before describing some of this work, however, let us examine in more detail the consequences of removing the thymus gland from both neonatal and adult animals.

Probably the most significant change associated with thymectomy is a depletion of the circulating pool of small lymphocytes. A deficiency of these cells occurs in the blood, thoracic duct lymph, and in those areas of the spleen and lymph nodes known to be traversed by the recirculating small lymphocytes on their way from blood to lymph, i.e., the so-called thymus-dependent areas. When the thymus is removed in neonatal mice, this depletion becomes evident at an early age, there being no appreciable postnatal increase in the number of recirculating cells. For example, in mice which have been sham-thymectomized at birth, the absolute lymphocyte count and the lymphocyte:polymorphonuclear ratio increases progressively during the first eight days of life, reaching almost the normal adult ratio. In neonatally thymectomized animals, however, there is no significant increase in this ratio. Indeed, cannulation of the thoracic ducts

* In a newborn mouse the thymus is about 3 mm long and 2 mm wide. The organ continues to enlarge until the age of weaning (three to four weeks); then it begins to decrease in size in the process known as age involution. This process occurs in all animals including man.

of six-week-old mice which have been thymectomized at birth reveals the output of lymphocytes during the first twenty-four to forty-eight hours of drainage to be only 1 to 3% of that of normal control mice of similar age and strain. On the other hand, when adult animals are thymectomized, there is only a gradual decline in the number of circulating pool small lymphocytes, the lowest levels being reached after several months, and there are no immediate immunological consequences. Thus when two-month-old rats are thymectomized, a period of more than two months is required for the lymphocyte content of the blood and thoracic duct to fall to 60% of normal levels. This lymphopenia can, however, be greatly accelerated and accentuated by whole-body X-irradiation. In fact, thymectomized adults which are subjected to lethal doses of irradiation (850 r) and saved by infusion of bone marrow cells, which re-equips them with erythropoietic and myelopoietic cells, remain lymphopenic and behave like neonatally thymectomized mice when challenged with skin grafts. These findings demonstrate that, not only does the thymus influence the development of the circulating pool small lymphocytes in early life, but it is also necessary to maintain their numbers throughout life.

Since, as we have already seen, circulating pool small lymphocytes include immunologically competent cells which are intimately involved in cell-mediated types of immune reactions, such as homograft rejection and delayed hypersensitivity reactions (see Chapter 8), a deficiency of these cells affects primarily this category of responses rather than those which are mediated by humoral antibodies. Indeed, the influence of the thymus on this latter class of immunological reactions is far from clear. All that is known is that it seems to vary according to the species, the time of antigen challenge, the nature of the antigen, and other factors pertaining to the immunization. For example, in some species neonatal thymectomy depresses the primary response to some antigens, whereas in others the primary response may be normal, or nearly normal, while the secondary response is delayed or significantly reduced in magnitude. Furthermore, neonatal thymectomy does not appear to have any significant effect on immunoglobulin levels, or on the type of immunoglobulin produced.

In the light of the above considerations it is not surprising that thymectomy has little or no effect on the development of cells of the lymphoid follicles and of plasma cells, i.e., cells responsible for immunoglobulin synthesis. This is particularly evident in chickens where there is another organ, the *bursa of Fabricius,* situated at the distal end of the intestinal tract just above the cloaca, which resembles the thymus in structure and appears to be necessary for the development of lymphoid follicles and plasma cells. Thus, chickens that have been bursectomized four days before hatching, or bursectomized and irradiated at hatching, have a normal complement of small lymphocytes and can reject skin transplants from other chickens in normal fashion. However, they are deficient in plasma cells and consequently fail completely to produce antibody in response to any of the standard antigens such as serum albumin or bacterial vaccines.*

As the original experiments of Miller and Martinez demonstrated, mice thymectomized at birth have a significantly impaired ability to reject skin homografts. Although the extent of this impairment is usually inversely related to the genetic disparity between the donor and the host, in some cases it is sufficient to prolong significantly the survival of *heterografts*. For example, Miller found that some neonatally thymectomized C3H mice accepted rat skin grafts for more than twenty-five days, a rather remarkable prolongation when one realizes that such grafts barely survive a week on normal recipients.

Cell-mediated reactions in other species may likewise be severely affected. For example, rats thymectomized at birth: (1) accept skin or tumor homografts for longer periods than normal littermates; (2) are more susceptible to graft-versus-host attack by homologous lymphoid cells; (3) give diminished, delayed hypersensitivity reactions to tuberculin; and (4) are less prone to develop autoallergic encephalomyelitis. Hamsters display an even greater degree of immunological impairment following thymectomy. This is evidenced by the observation that, when this organ is removed as late as two weeks after birth, the life expectancy of mouse skin heterografts may be prolonged by a factor of four. On the other hand, puppies thymectomized at birth are able to manifest a normal response when subsequently challenged with kidney homografts. This, of course, is due to the fact that in the dog, as in many other species, the state of lymphoid development is so well advanced at birth that homograft reactivity prevails, at least for a time, independently of the presence of a thymus as it does in rodents thymectomized in adult life.

Mice thymectomized at birth develop normally for the first few weeks. After weaning, however, many die from an acute wasting disease characterized clinically by weight loss, hunched posture, ruffled fur, and diarrhea. Autopsy reveals an extreme atrophy of the lymphoid organs.

---

* In chickens there appear to be two "central lymphoid organs": (1) the bursa of Fabricius which is responsible for the development of large lymphocytes and plasma cells essential for immunoglobulin synthesis and (2) the thymus, which controls the development of the small lymphocytes which mediate cellular immunities. Hence the question arises whether there is a bursal equivalent in mammals. In this regard, Dr. Robert Good and his colleagues have suggested that the appendix of the rabbit may represent a homologue of the bursa and that the mammalian tonsil and other lympho-epithelial tissues of the gastrointestinal tract, e.g., Peyer's patches, may subserve the functions of the bursa of Fabricius in other mammals, including man.

In general, the earlier in life thymectomy is performed, the higher the incidence of this syndrome, which does not occur in animals thymectomized after one week of age. There is also a great deal of interstrain variation in the onset of the disease. Some strains develop symptoms as early as four weeks of age, while others appear normal until they are four months old. A similar syndrome occurs in rats and hamsters which are thymectomized at birth.

Although this wasting disease has obvious resemblances to the syndromes seen in graft-versus-host conditions, such as runt disease in infant mice, secondary disease in radiation chimeras, F_1 hybrid disease, and parabiosis intoxication (see Chapter 11), its etiology is completely different. This is best exemplified by the fact that, whereas the graft-versus-host syndrome develops in both conventional and germ-free mice inoculated at birth with homologous cells, the wasting syndrome which follows neonatal thymectomy does *not* occur in germ-free animals. Indeed, neonatally thymectomized mice raised under germ-free conditions display no significant weight loss and do not differ in size from untreated and partially thymectomized littermates. The primary factor responsible for the pathogenesis of the postneonatal thymectomy wasting syndrome thus appears to be an environmental factor, presumably an infectious agent (or its product), to which only neonatally thymectomized mice, because of their reduced immunological capacity, are particularly susceptible.*

Prevention of Immunological Debilitating Effects of Neonatal Thymectomy

The effects of neonatal thymectomy can be prevented or reversed in a number of ways. For example, if 5 to 10 $\times$ 10^6 isologous adult spleen or lymph node cells are given to infant mice within a week after removal of

* It should be noted that, inasmuch as germ-free mice have a reduced total circulating lymphocyte pool to begin with, neonatal thymectomy does not accentuate this situation nor does it decrease the already sparse cellularity of the lymphoid tissues. However, germ-free mice thymectomized at birth, in contrast to normal germ-free animals, display a depressed response to sheep erythrocytes very similar to that seen in conventional neonatally thymectomized subjects. They also accept skin homografts for prolonged periods, but not as long as in conventionally thymectomized animals. This latter situation may stem from the fact that, under normal conditions, a higher proportion of the available antigen-sensitive cells in an already limited pool may become committed to bacterial antigens, or, put another way, in the absence of bacterial contamination, more cells may be available to react against a skin homograft.

their thymus, wasting disease does not occur and homograft reactivity is restored in the majority of subjects. This reconstitution undoubtedly occurs because these suspensions include cells which, having already attained immunological competence, can equip their thymectomized hosts with a functional lymphoid system. Suspensions of isologous thymocytes can also reverse the effects of thymectomy but only if given in amounts twenty to forty times in excess of the required number of adult splenic or lymph node cells. This is likewise consistent with their providing immunologically competent cells, as only a small fraction of "thymocytes" are known to function in this capacity. Whether these cells are derived from within the substance of the thymus de novo or whether they have migrated into the thymus from the peripheral lymphoid tissues remains to be determined.

The immunological deficiency of neonatally thymectomized mice can also be prevented by grafts or implants of whole lobes of thymus tissue placed either subcutaneously or under the renal capsule. Thus when mice that have been thymectomized at birth receive, within three or four weeks, grafts of thymic tissue from donor mice of the same strain, they do not develop the wasting syndrome, their lymphoid organs produce lymphocytes at about the normal rate, and they are fully capable of undertaking cell-mediated immune reactions. When the donor and host are of *different,* but H-2 compatible, strains, the host is incapable of rejecting skin grafts from either strain, though it rejects third-party skin grafts normally.

While the obvious explanation for the protection afforded by these thymic implants is that they are producing lymphocytes which colonize the lymphoid tissues of the thymectomized host, the experimental evidence is not completely in accord with this interpretation. For example, if neonatally thymectomized mice are subsequently restored by a subcutaneous thymus graft composed of cells which are chromosomally "tagged," the majority of cells which are eventually found in both the host lymphoid tissues and the thymus graft are not of graft but of *host* origin. Similar results have likewise been reported in man. When two male infants suffering from a congenital absence of the thymus * were treated with female

* In 1965 DiGeorge described infants with a congenital absence of the organs embryologically derived from the third and fourth pharyngeal pouches—the thymus and parathyroid glands. This presented a unique opportunity for evaluating the role of the thymus in man. Other cases of what is now known as DiGeorge's Syndrome have subsequently been reported. In these infants, as in neonatally thymectomized mice, cell-mediated immunity is severely impaired. They are incapable of manifesting delayed hypersensitivity reactions and accept skin homografts indefinitely or for greatly prolonged periods. On the other hand, humoral immunity is intact (cortical germinal centers and medullary plasma cells are normal). It is therefore evident that the dichotomy found between cellular and humoral immunity in laboratory animals also occurs in man.

thymic fragments implanted in their rectus abdominis muscle, the immediate increase in circulating lymphocytes which they displayed proved, on cytological analysis, to be of host (XY) rather than of graft (XX) genotype.

It therefore appears that these thymic implants are effective, not by actually contributing cells, but by either producing some noncellular factor which stimulates lymphopoiesis or by providing an environment suitable for lymphoid cell differentiation.

To explore this problem, an ingenious series of experiments was carried out by Osoba and Miller, in England, and by Levey, Trainin, and Law at the National Institutes of Health. Osoba and Miller implanted into the peritoneal cavity of week-old mice, which had been thymectomized at birth, Millipore diffusion chambers containing embryonic thymus tissue. The pore size of these chambers did not permit the passage of intact cells but did allow their products to pass into the host. The subsequent growth of these mice was normal, and when they were challenged with skin homografts, their survival times fell within the normal range. Nevertheless, most of these animals did display some diminution in the population of lymphocytes in both blood and tissues. When the Millipore chambers were recovered after one to two months, they contained only epithelial-reticular cells and no lymphoid cells.

Similar findings were reported by the Bethesda group, who also removed the thymus from mice soon after birth but waited three to four weeks before implanting into the abdominal cavity a diffusion chamber containing a whole thymus taken from a newborn donor mouse of the same strain. These animals also grew and survived almost like normal animals. Their body weight increased steadily; they showed no signs of wasting disease and were immunologically competent. Moreover, in contrast to the findings of Osoba and Miller, these investigators found no depletion of lymphocytes in either the solid tissues or the blood. In summary, thymectomized animals which received thymus tissue enclosed in Millipore chambers did about as well as those which received it subcutaneously or under the kidney capsule.

These experiments indicated that thymic tissue can elaborate a diffusible agent that acts on lymphoid precursor cells present in neonatally thymectomized mice, causing them to differentiate and mature into immunologically competent cells. Subsequent work yielded results consistent with this thesis. For example, it was found that, after neonatally thymectomized female mice had a litter, they displayed a normal ability to respond to skin homografts. Since later experiments ruled out the possibilities that this regained competence was due to a sex hormonal influence or to fetal lymphoid cells traversing the placenta and "seeding" maternal lymphoid tissue, the most likely explanation was that a thymus-derived humoral factor produced by the fetuses gained access to the maternal circulation and stimulated lymphocytopoiesis. Finally, Law has had some success in preventing wasting disease, and in restoring the immunological capacities of neonatally thymectomized mice, by implanting into their dorsal subcutaneous tissue, within twenty-four hours of thymectomy, one lobe of a neonatal rat or hamster thymus. Since only epithelial-reticular cells persisted in these heterografts, it seems most likely that some humoral factor produced by these cells was responsible for the restoration observed.*

The fact that a thymus hormone is apparently necessary to convert lymphoid precursor cells into immunologically competent cells does not negate the possibility that the thymus is also the source of these precursor cells. Indeed, there are some grounds for believing that the restoration of neonatally thymectomized animals with thymus grafts sequestered in diffusion chambers results from the action of a hormone released from these chambers upon cells which escaped from the host's thymus before it was removed. Recent studies in which lymphocytes were labeled intrathymically in newborn rats indicate that a considerable portion of the total lymphocyte population of the spleen and lymph nodes is derived from the thymus. It therefore seems reasonable to assume that at least some of these cells migrate from this gland before parturition. Osoba's and Miller's observation that neonatally thymectomized mice remain lymphocytopenic even after their immunological competence has been restored with chambers containing thymus tissue is also in accord with this view.

Origin of Thymic Lymphocytes

The origin of thymic lymphocytes has also been a matter of conjecture. Initially it was believed, mainly on the basis of in vitro experiments, that these cells were derived from the epithelial cells of the organ anlage. However, all the evidence now suggests that they originate from blood-borne cells which are only able to proliferate and differentiate into lymphoid cells under the influence of thymic epithelial cells. The most convincing series of experiments in this regard has been carried out by J. J. T. Owen

---

* More recently, Abraham White and his associates at Albert Einstein College of Medicine in New York have isolated and partially purified a soluble lymphocytopoietic factor, known as *thymosin*, from calf thymus. When given to normal mice, this factor stimulates lymphocytopoiesis as reflected by an increase in peripheral lymphoid tissue weight and augmented incorporation of labeled precursors into the DNA and protein of lymphoid cells. Thymosin also accelerates lymphoid tissue regeneration in mice exposed to whole-body X-irradiation. In neonatally thymectomized mice, thymosin restores immunological competence to spleen cells and reduces the incidence of wasting disease. The relationship between thymosin and the humoral factor produced by isologous, homologous, or heterologous thymic implants remains to be determined.

and his associates at Oxford. For example, they found that, if thymic rudiments from chick or mouse embryos are cultured in diffusion chambers on the chick chorioallantois, where their supply of blood-borne cells is cut off, rudiments from older embryos become fully lymphoid whereas primordia from early embryos fail to develop lymphoid cells. By selecting rudiments from embryos of various ages, they were able to demonstrate that blood-derived stem cells first enter the chick thymic anlage at between six and seven days of incubation and the mouse thymic rudiment, between ten and eleven days of gestation.

A blood-borne origin for thymic lymphocytes is also in accord with evidence which suggests that in adult animals these cells are derived from hemopoietic tissue. For example, by means of chromosome marker techniques it can be shown that, when marrow cells are injected into X-irradiated mice, they proliferate initially in both marrow and thymus, whereas injected thymus and lymph node cells proliferate only in lymph nodes. The cells which proliferate in the thymus have all the characteristics of thymic cells. Moreover, the cells bearing the marker of the injected thymus and lymph node cells completely disappear after a period of time and are replaced by cells bearing the marrow marker, which become present throughout. These findings indicate that the irradiated thymus receives cells from the bone marrow and that it induces these cells to differentiate along lymphoid pathways. They likewise suggest that throughout the life of normal animals there is an inward afferent stream of cells entering the intact thymus, as well as a natural efferent flow of cells which leave this organ for sites of lymphoid tissue elsewhere in the body. Although it has yet to be proven, at least some of these cells which leave the thymus may be those with a long life span which make an important contribution to the pool of small lymphocytes outside the thymus. If this is so, it would explain why the immunologically competent cells of neonatally thymectomized animals or of athymic infants restored with thymus grafts are of *host* origin, i.e., they would represent stem cells derived from the hemopoietic tissue of the host which, under the influence of the thymus graft, differentiate into cells capable of mediating cellular immunities.

The Thymus and Immunologic Tolerance

Finally, there is also evidence which suggests that the thymus, because of the influence it exerts on the differentiation of new, immunologically competent cells, plays a role in breaking down artificially induced immunological tolerance (see Chapter 10), and that it may be directly involved in the induction of tolerance as well. Evidence for the former comes from these facts:

1. Mice rendered immunologically tolerant of protein antigens by exposure from birth to adulthood lose their tolerance at a significantly slower rate after injections are stopped if they have been thymectomized as adults.

2. The transplantation of isologous thymus tissue to mice tolerant of skin homografts accelerates the abolition of tolerance.

The importance of the thymus in the induction of tolerance is indicated by a series of experiments carried out by Toullet and Waksman. These investigators grafted three-week-old, neonatally thymectomized, strain A mice with a single thymus from either a normal strain A donor or one which had been rendered tolerant at birth of CBA antigens. Whereas those which received the normal thymus graft showed a nearly normal ability to reject CBA skin, recipients of thymuses from tolerant donors were specifically tolerant of CBA skin grafts.

It is evident that the surface has only been scratched in elucidating the role which the thymus plays in the development of competence to undertake cellular immunities. Nevertheless, it already is clear that its function bears directly on transplantation immunity and tolerance, on the etiology of autoimmune diseases, and on the development of neoplasias.

REFERENCES

Beard, J. 1899. The true function of the thymus. Lancet. i:144–146.

Good, R. A., and A. E. Gabrielsen [ed.]. 1964. The thymus in immunobiology. Hoeber and Row, New York.

Defendi, V., and D. Metcalf [ed.]. 1964. The thymus. Wistar Inst. Symp. Monog. No. 2. Wistar Press, Philadelphia.

Metcalf, D. 1966. The thymus. *In* Recent results in cancer research. Monog. No. 5. Springer-Verlag, New York.

Miller, J. F. A. P., and D. Osoba. 1967. Current concepts of the immunological function of the thymus. Physiol. Rev. 47:437–520.

Miller, J. F. A. P. 1967. The thymus yesterday, today, and tomorrow. Lancet, ii:1299–1302.

Miller, J. F. A. P., and G. F. Mitchell. 1969. Thymus and antigen-reactive cells. Transpl. Rev. 1:3–42. Munksgaard, Copenhagen, Denmark.

Chapter 10

Immunological Tolerance

Immunologists have long been aware that inoculation of embryos or very young animals with antigens usually fails to incite any perceptible response. From this, they very reasonably concluded that such recipients were too immature to undertake any kind of reaction. We now know that this is not the case, for when embryos or young animals are inoculated with an antigenic substance they may be so affected that, when they grow up, their capacity to respond to that antigen is weakened or totally suppressed. This state of specific immunological inactivity is known as *immunological tolerance,* and the important clue which led to its discovery was provided by a condition which arises naturally in cattle.

When unlike-sexed twins occur in cattle, the male is usually completely normal, but his female co-twin is often a modified, sterile female known as a *freemartin.* The external genitalia of these animals are female, but the internal sex organs and their accessories are more or less male-like, varying from one individual to another. Because these females represent genetic females which have developed in a male direction, they attracted the attention of embryologists and endocrinologists concerned with the problem of sex differentiation. Thus, as long ago as 1916, Professor F. R. Lillie demonstrated that, in order for the freemartin condition to occur, there had to be an anastomosis of blood vessels between the chorions of the dissimilar bovine twin embryos. From this he concluded that hormones of the male twin, having gained access to the circulation of its female co-twin, diverted the normal development of her sex apparatus. This interpretation led to many frustrating attempts by Lillie and his students to reproduce with the appropriate hormones, in a variety of laboratory animals, what had been accomplished by Nature in the freemartin. We are now aware that these failures were at least partly due to the fact that freemartins not only possess male hormones but male cells as well. This was demonstrated in 1945 by Ray D. Owen who showed that, as a result of a natural prenatal exchange of red-cell precursors, most twin cattle are born with, and may retain throughout life, a stable though variable mixture of each other's erythrocytes, i.e., they are *chimeras*. This discovery was followed a few years later by Burnet's and Fenner's theory of antibody formation. This theory, greatly influenced by Owen's finding, predicted that, if embryos are exposed to antigenic substances, their ability to react against these same substances when they grow up would be abolished or at least impaired.

Shortly thereafter, Medawar and his associates showed that most dizygotic cattle twins would accept skin grafts from each other but not from their parents or siblings of separate birth or from unrelated third parties. This observation emerged from work which had been initiated with the mistaken belief that monozygotic and dizygotic twins in cattle could be distinguished according to the fate of skin grafts exchanged between them, as they can in man and in most other species. Once the connection between Owen's discovery of chimerism and this observation of homograft survival was realized, the stage was set to reproduce in the laboratory the state of affairs that occurs as a natural accident in twin cattle *

Experimental Induction of Tolerance in Young Animals

The initial attempts to produce tolerant animals experimentally stemmed from the independent efforts of Medawar and his associates in

* Erythrocyte chimerism is not limited to twins, triplets, etc., in cattle but occurs in other species as well. For example, in marmosets, chimerism resulting from vascular anastomoses between the placentae of twins is very frequent, although unaccompanied by any influence on sex. Its occurrence in sheep and man is rare. In man, only nine cases have thus far been reported. In many of these animals, chimerism has been demonstrated by means of sex-chromatin or sex-chromosome analyses of peripheral blood leukocytes, and tolerance has been confirmed by acceptance of the appropriate skin grafts. Note that vascular anastomosis does not necessarily result in the exchange of only hematopoietic cells—other cells are exchanged as well. Indeed, as more recent evidence indicates, it seems likely that the sex modification which occurs in the freemartin is due to the transfer of cellular components of male gonadal tissue rather than hormones. Finally, there is also evidence that the relative proportions of the two antigenically distinct types of cells in cattle chimeric twins may change with time and that "hybrid" type erythrocytes may appear. Thus, Stone and his colleagues at the University of Wisconsin have reported a case where the blood of one chimeric twin, which at three years of age contained two red-cell types, 10% representing his own genotype and 90% the genotype of his co-twin, at eight years of age had three blood types, the two parental types, each representing 2%, and a "hybrid" type representing 96% of the cell population. It is believed that the "hybrid" cell type, which presumably must have had a distinct selective advantage, resulted from "matings" between the two genetically distinct types of hematopoietic stem cells present.

London, and of Hašek in Prague (see Fig. 10.1). The former group of investigators inoculated CBA mouse embryos of about fifteen or sixteen days of age (the gestation period of the mouse is about twenty days) with a viable suspension of adult tissue cells derived from strain A mice. This cell suspension, which originated from testis, kidney, and splenic tissue, was introduced directly into each fetus through a very fine hypodermic needle. Eight weeks after they were born, and at a time when they were

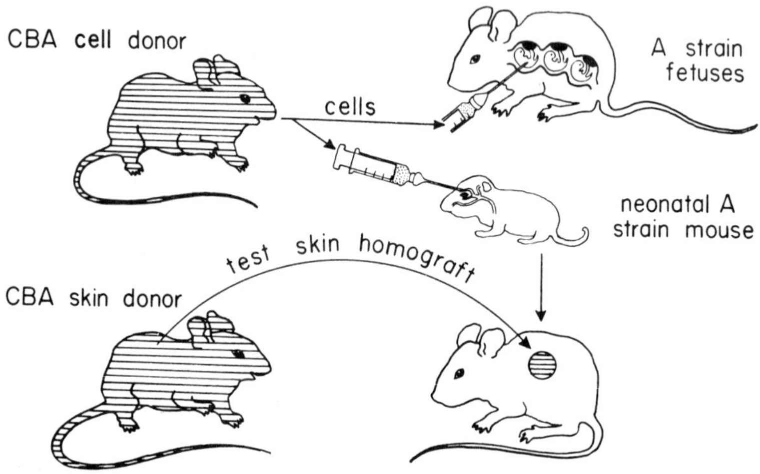

Fig. 10.1. Methods of inducing tolerance of CBA skin grafts in A strain mice. A cell suspension, usually prepared from the spleen of an adult CBA mouse, is inoculated either into strain A fetuses or, intravenously, into newborn strain A mice. Such treated mice accept CBA skin homografts when adult.

immunologically competent, these animals were challenged with strain A skin grafts which either were permanently accepted or survived for a significantly longer period of time than similar grafts on untreated CBA hosts. The tolerance so induced was specific since animals rendered unresponsive to A strain tissues rejected homografts from the unrelated AU strain.*

Similar results were also obtained in White Leghorn chickens given intravenous injections of blood from Rhode Island Red embryos on the

---

* If, however, the second donor strain happens to share some important antigens in common with the donor which provided the tolerance-conferring inoculum, a skin graft from this second donor strain may display prolonged survival. For example, if A strain mice made fully tolerant of C3H strain skin homografts by inoculation with C3H cells at birth are challenged with CBA strain homografts (of the same H-2 genotype as C3H), the latter survive for about twenty-four days instead of eleven days as on normal A strain hosts.

eleventh or twelfth day of incubation. Of course, in this instance the success of the experiments was dependent upon the strict pairing of donors and recipients, i.e., chicks exposed to blood from one Rhode Island Red donor did not display tolerance of skin grafts obtained from another member of the same breed since the donor breed was comprised of a genetically heterogeneous group of animals.

Hašek also reproduced Owen's phenomenon in chickens but utilized a different model system. His system was based on procuring synchorial parabiosis of avian embryos by approximation of the highly vascular chorioallantoic membranes which are located beneath the shells. Through the vascular anastomoses that become established, an intensive exchange of blood between both partners takes place, just as it does naturally in the case of cattle twins. When these parabiotic pairs were hatched, they were found incapable of producing isoagglutinins when challenged with erythrocytes from their partners. They also accepted grafts of their partners' skin.

These experiments confirmed the predictions of Burnet's and Fenner's theory of immunity. They also initiated a whole new field of immunology, a field which has been especially significant insofar as tissue transplantation is concerned and, consequently, one which has grown almost logarithmically over the past decade and a half.

When the phenomenon of tolerance was first discovered, it was generally believed that tolerance could be induced only during a finite period of life, which varied from species to species in accordance with the degree of maturity of the fetuses at term. This period became known as the *tolerance-responsive period* and was thought to terminate well before birth in cattle, sheep, man, and other mammals with relatively long gestation periods; at or just after term in rabbits, mice, and chickens; and within the first two weeks of life in rats and ducks. Moreover, since it was apparent that the same antigenic stimulus that induced unresponsiveness in embryos or young animals caused older recipients to become sensitized or immune, it was also believed that there must be a gradual transition from one modality of response to the other. On this basis the existence of a second period, the so-called neutral or "null period," was also postulated, i.e., an age or age-range at which exposure to an antigen conferred neither tolerance or immunity. In the light of subsequent findings, however, especially those which demonstrated that tolerance was not the prerogative of young, immunologically immature animals (under certain conditions, discussed below, adult animals can frequently be rendered unresponsive to homografts), it became evident that neither of these concepts could be sustained in their original sense. Thus, although the term "tolerance-responsive period" is useful operationally to designate the age range at which tolerance is *readily* induced by exposure to antigen, it doesn't imply the existence of a period beyond which tolerance induction is impossible. Furthermore, the termination of such a period varies inversely with the immunogenetic disparity between donor and host. For example, in mice, tolerance of H-2 antigens can be induced readily only if the homologous cells are introduced no later than a few hours after birth, at which time it is almost obligatory that they be given intravenously.* This is usually accomplished via the orbital branch of the anterior facial vein. On the other hand, tolerance of the Y antigen in female C57BL/6 mice can be easily achieved as late as seventeen days postpartum, irrespective of the route in which the isologous cells are presented (see Table 10.1).

Table 10.1

Induction of tolerance in C57BL/6 female mice by inoculation with isologous male spleen cells. Mice 12 days of age, or less, received 5–10 million cells, and older animals received 12–20 million. All tolerant animals bore perfect male skin isografts for upwards of 150 days. (sc = subcutaneous; iv = intravenous; ip = intraperitoneal route of injection.)

Age at injection	*Route*	*Number of mice tested*	*Tolerant (%)*
< 24 hours	sc	5	100
< 24 hours	iv	20	100
4 days	iv	6	100
4 days	ip	9	100
6 days	ip	9	100
12 days	ip	14	93
17 days	ip	15	60
21 days	ip	23	9

The initial studies on immunological tolerance also suggested that cells of different origins were equally effective in inducing tolerance and that no tissue specificity was involved. That is, mice or rats inoculated at birth with

* Indeed, with some H-2 incompatible donor/recipient combinations, it is virtually impossible to induce tolerance even in newborn hosts merely by inoculating homologous cells. Thus although twenty million (C57BL × A) F_1 hybrid spleen cells—about the maximum number of cells that can safely be administered intravenously to a neonatal mouse—will render about 10% of C57BL mice partially tolerant of A strain skin, none of these grafts survive for fifty days. However, this apparent refractoriness of neonatal C57BL mice to the induction of tolerance can easily be overcome by exposing them to a sublethal dosage of X-irradiation (about 300 r) before inoculation of the cellular antigen. Following this treatment, the majority of the subjects display high degrees of tolerance of A strain skin grafts.

cell suspensions derived from a variety of organs including bone marrow, spleen, lymph nodes, blood, and mammary tumors become completely tolerant of skin and other tissues—adrenal cortex, ovary, thyroid, parathyroid, kidney, etc. These conclusions, too, have had to be modified. We now know that there are wide disparities in the tolerance-inducing efficacy of cells of different origin. Moreover, this may vary from species to species and is again influenced by the genetic disparity between donor and host. For example, in mice, an extensive series of tests conducted with the H-2 incompatible CBA $\longrightarrow$ A strain combination revealed that, at similar dosage levels, lymph node cells were most effective in inducing tolerance of CBA skin grafts. Blood leukocytes and splenic cells were about equally effective, being demonstrably inferior to node cells, but significantly superior to marrow cells, and thymocytes were least effective of all the inocula tested (Fig. 10.2). On the other hand, in rats, tolerance of Ag-B antigens is most easily accomplished with bone marrow cells. Indeed, spleen and node cells are very ineffective in inducing tolerance of Ag-B incompatible skin grafts, and thymocytes are even worse.*

While it is difficult to understand why cell suspensions of similar genetic origin differ in their capacity to induce tolerance of skin homografts in mice and rats, recent results obtained with the latter species suggest that animals inoculated at birth with Ag-B incompatible lymph node cells may be rendered tolerant of these cells but *not* of skin grafts of the same genetic origin. Thus BN rats inoculated at birth with (Lewis × BN) F_1 hybrid lymph node cells may reject Lewis skin grafts with the vigor and promptitude of normal animals, even though their blood lymphocytes are comparatively unreactive to (Lewis × BN) F_1 lymphocytes in culture† (see Chapter 8). The basis for this paradox is unknown. One possibility is that, when Ag-B incompatibility prevails, bone marrow (which is the most effective source of cells for rendering neonatal rats highly tolerant of subsequent skin grafts) and skin cells share an antigen(s) which is poorly represented on lymph node cells. A complete absence on lymph node cells of one or more of the important Ag-B antigenic specificities present on skin and marrow cells seems improbable since neonatal rats inoculated with high dosages ($\geqq 30 \times 10^6$) of lymph node cells occasionally do become permanently tolerant of skin grafts.

A deficiency of one or more of the Ag-B specificities present in marrow, lymph node, and skin cells seems a more likely explanation for the

* It should be noted, however, that lymph node cells and thymocytes are effective in inducing high degrees of tolerance of subsequent skin grafts when donor and host are Ag-B compatible.

† Lymphocytes from BN rats inoculated neonatally with Lewis bone marrow cells are also unreactive to (BN × Lewis) F_1 lymphocytes in culture.

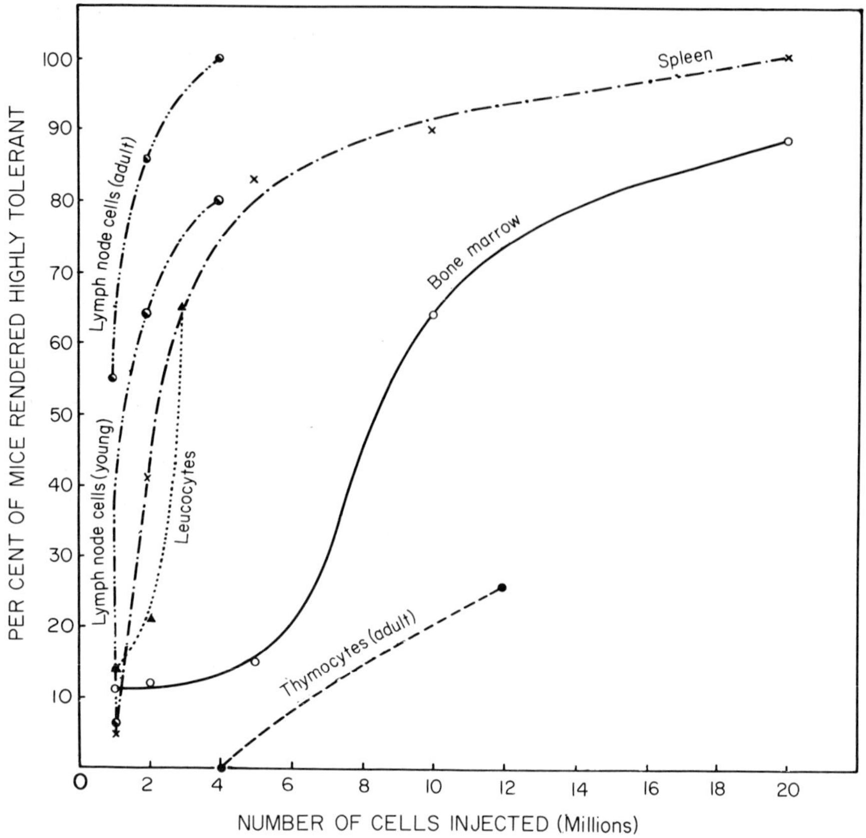

Fig. 10.2. Curves showing percentages of A strain mice made highly tolerant of CBA skin grafts following their intravenous inoculation at birth with various dosages of living cell suspensions of different histological origins prepared from CBA strain donors. "Highly tolerant" refers to the acceptance of a CBA skin graft for at least fifty days. Note that lymph node cells constitute the most effective tolerance-conferring inoculum, that leukocytes and splenic cells are next, being demonstrably better than bone marrow cells, and that thymocytes are least effective.

tolerogenic inadequacy of rat thymocytes, since lymphocytes from rats inoculated at birth with thymocytes are fully reactive in vitro, and high degrees of tolerance of skin grafts have never been induced with these cells.

The following observations are also consistent with the fact that animals chimeric with regard to cells of one tissue need not necessarily be tolerant of cells from another tissue of the same genetic origin:

1. If newborn strain A mice are inoculated with (C57BL × CBA) F_1 hybrid spleen or marrow cells, the survivors may be only moderately tolerant of hybrid or C57BL skin grafts, yet may display a much higher degree of tolerance of subsequent CBA grafts, so that the latter outlive

those from C57BL donors. This is known as *split tolerance*. Chimera tests on such animals indicate that they contain foreign cells bearing both CBA and C57BL antigens, even *after* they have rejected C57BL or hybrid skin grafts. For example, suspensions of spleen cells prepared from such animals confer a perceptible tolerance of CBA skin on inoculation into neonatal strain A hosts.

2. Dizygotic cattle twins with erythrocyte chimerism may exhibit complete tolerance of each other's hematopoietic tissues and, at the same time, be incompletely tolerant of skin grafts. Thus Stone and his colleagues have reported that skin grafts exchanged between partners of twenty-one pairs of chimeric twins were rejected by more than half of the twins in an average of 250 days. A similar situation has also been reported in man. Woodruff and Lennox exchanged skin grafts between a pair of human bisexual red-cell chimeric twins. Whereas one twin appeared completely tolerant of its test graft throughout the six-month observation period, suggestive evidence was obtained of cellular replacement in the graft on the other twin, which the investigators consider indicative of partial tolerance. However, there was no change in the proportion of foreign erythrocytes in the blood of either twin.

3. Finally, there is evidence that donor-type γ-globulins may be found in homologous mouse radiation chimeras (see Chapter 11) despite the fact that donor-type skin homografts are rejected.

It should also be noted that transplantation tolerance can only be consistently conferred by inoculation of cells of the erythropoietic, myeloid, or lymphoid series. With other types of cells, successes have been very fitful even when minor histoincompatibilities prevail and high-dosage inocula are employed.* Thus, whereas even thymocytes are highly effective in inducing tolerance of skin in Ag-B compatible neonatal rats (but *not* in Ag-B incompatible animals), epidermal cell suspensions and cell suspensions prepared from adult kidney, liver, testis, etc., are ineffective. Moreover, no one has been able to induce tolerance of skin with cells which have been propagated in vitro. Exposure of cells to irradiation also impairs or abolishes their tolerance-conferring capacity, and few successes have attended attempts to make neonatal animals tolerant by inoculation with antigenic extracts. The relative inability of cells from nonlymphohematopoietic organ sources, irradiated cells, or antigenic extracts to induce tolerance in newborn animals is almost certainly due to their failure to

* The original attempts of Billingham, Brent, and Medawar to induce tolerance by inoculating a suspension of cells derived from spleen, kidney, and testis would probably have been unsuccessful if spleen cells had been omitted.

migrate, proliferate, and become permanently established in the host's seats of immunological response.

Apart from the type of cell in an inoculum, the *dosage* of cells is likewise an important factor in determining whether tolerance will be conferred and whether it will be complete or partial. As might be expected, the number of cells required to induce tolerance is much greater when donor and host differ at a major histocompatibility locus than when differences at only nonmajor loci are involved. Indeed, when a major histocompatibility difference exists, small numbers of cells may induce immunity rather than unresponsiveness. Thus, if Lewis rats are inoculated at birth with 10^5 BN bone marrow cells, or A strain mice are given a neonatal, intraperitoneal inoculation of 2×10^5 (CBA $\times$ A) F_1 hybrid spleen cells, they respond in an immune manner when subsequently challenged with the appropriate skin graft.

The Abolition of Tolerance

All the evidence presented so far suggests that tolerance represents a specific failure of the host's immunological response mechanism, i.e., an adaptation to the antigen on the part of the *host*. But this does not entirely rule out the possibility that the homologous cells which induce tolerance, as well as skin and other organ homografts which have been in residence in tolerant animals for long periods, also undergo some kind of antigenic change or adaptation. That this does not occur is indicated by the fact that, if skin homografts which have been maintained on tolerant animals for prolonged periods are removed and returned to their strain of origin, they are permanently accepted, whereas if they are transplanted to a normal (i.e., nontolerant) member of the same strain on which they have been in residence, they are promptly rejected. Further evidence against the adaptation of tolerated grafts also derives from the following simple experiment. If an A strain mouse bearing a healthy CBA skin homograft of long standing (as a result of neonatal inoculation with CBA spleen cells) is injected with lymph node or splenic cells from a normal A strain mouse which has *itself* been actively immunized against CBA tissue, the hitherto tolerated graft will begin to deteriorate within a short period of time, and breakdown is soon complete. This indicates not only that the antigenicity of the tolerated graft has remained unchanged, but also that a tolerant animal is perfectly capable of implementing an immunity of *adoptive* origin (see Chapter 8).

If, instead of implanting the tolerant A strain mouse with *sensitized* lymphoid cells from an actively immunized animal of its own strain, it is inoculated with normal lymphoid cells from an untreated A strain donor, breakdown of the tolerated graft still takes place, though the process is much slower. This experiment shows that the foreign cells present in the tolerant mouse must have been producing (and possibly liberating) antigens all the time, but that the host was unable to recognize them as such. When normal, immunologically competent cells from an isologous donor are introduced into a tolerant mouse, they respond to these antigens with the result that the graft and presumably all the established cells of the neonatal inoculum as well are destroyed.*

Induction of Tolerance in Adult Animals

Contrary to what was originally believed when the phenomenon was first discovered, tolerance of tissue homografts can also be induced in adult mice. This usually requires their exposure to massive amounts of antigen over prolonged periods. It may be effected by *repeated* injections of very high dosages of homologous cells, or by maintaining the intended host in parabiotic union with a partner which provides the appropriate cellular antigens with respect to which unresponsiveness is to be induced. The magnitude and duration of the exposure necessary to induce tolerance in these immunologically mature animals again depends upon the degree of genetic disparity between donor and host. When they are very similar, short periods of parabiosis, or even a single, high dosage inoculum of homologous cells, may suffice; but when the differences involve more powerful antigens, heroic procedures are usually necessary.

To give some examples: A high proportion of adult C57BL females are rendered highly tolerant of the relatively weak Y antigen following

---

* This ability to transfer sensitivity adoptively to tolerant mice and rats bearing long-established skin homografts represents a very sensitive and objective assay system for investigating the immunological competence of cells of different origin. It also represents a means of determining the importance of other factors, e.g., humoral antibodies, in mediating homograft sensitivity. Thus, by means of this test system, it has been shown that in mice immunologically activated cells, capable of transferring homograft sensitivity, are present in the blood, peritoneal exudates, thoracic duct, spleen, and regional nodes of animals which have rejected skin homografts. Moreover, with this system it has also been shown that, when animals are sensitized with skin homografts, but *not* by means of splenic cell suspensions inoculated intraperitoneally, activated cells are highly persistent, still being demonstrable in both the blood and nodes more than a year after sensitization. Finally, in ducks and rats, some success has attended attempts to abolish tolerance with hyperimmune serum, although, at least with respect to the latter species, this loss of tolerance is presumed to be due mainly to a loss of cellular chimerism (see Chapter 7).

an intravenous or intraperitoneal inoculation of about 500×10^6 isologous male spleen cells (dosages within the range 2 to 100×10^6 sensitize the hosts). The intravenous route is the most effective, and *repeated* exposure to male cells is better than a single exposure. Such females also become unresponsive following about three weeks of parabiotic union with isologous males. The demanding nature of the treatments needed to induce tolerance in adults is indicated by the fact that similar degrees of tolerance can be induced in *neonatal* females by exposing them to as few as 2.5×10^4 isologous male spleen cells.

With the A $\longrightarrow$ C3H strain combination, which involves an H-2 difference, tolerance of skin grafts can consistently be obtained by intravenous and intraperitoneal (but not just intraperitoneal) injection of *adult* recipients, over a period of seven weeks, with a total number of about 1.5×10^9 (A $\times$ C3H) F_1 hybrid splenic cells. Similar degrees of unresponsiveness can also be induced if C3H adults are parabiotically united with (A $\times$ C3H) F_1 hybrids for thirty to forty-five days. Again, some indication of the massive antigenic exposure which is necessary to induce unresponsiveness in these adult recipients is given by the fact that high degrees of tolerance of strain A skin grafts can be obtained in about 50% of C3H animals if they are inoculated at birth with ten million (A $\times$ C3H) F_1 splenic cells.

The induction of unresponsiveness in adult animals can be facilitated by treatment with a number of immunosuppressive agents such as purine and pyrimidine antagonists, sublethal X-irradiation, thoracic duct drainage, antilymphocyte serum, etc. The use of such agents in some exact temporal relation to the administration of antigen results in tolerance under circumstances in which the antigen alone would produce an immune response (see Chapter 13). For example, Delta Uphoff has induced tolerance in mice of subsequent H-2 compatible skin grafts by pretreatment with A-methopterin or 6-mercaptopurine (6-MP), together with splenic and thymus cell inocula of appropriate origin. Tolerance was achieved only after the drug and cells were administered at high levels for considerable periods. Similarly, Anne McLaren found that, whereas 6-MP administration to adult mice for two weeks at near lethal doses significantly prolonged the survival of a proportion of homologous skin grafts, it did not induce permanent immunological tolerance. However, if, following 6-MP treatment, homologous spleen cell suspensions were given, permanent tolerance to a subsequent skin graft resulted, provided that donors and recipients belonged to the same H-2 group. Even more dramatic results have been obtained with mice treated with methylhydrazine derivatives—drugs which appear selectively to destroy lymphoid cells—and donor spleen cells. The daily administration of these drugs for three to four weeks prior to test grafting, combined with the intravenous inoculation of from 45 to 65×10^6 CBA spleen cells twelve or one days before transplantation, resulted in permanent tolerance of CBA skin grafts in about 30% of H-2 incompatible A strain recipients.

Michie and Woodruff also found that the ability of adult A strain mice to reject CBA grafts can be specifically inhibited by prior exposure to 350 to 400 r, followed by injection with 0.7-1.2 × 10^9 (CBA × A) F_1 splenic cells administered by both the intravenous and intraperitoneal routes. The principal function of irradiation here is probably to liberate sites for colonization by the inoculated cells, rather than to destroy the host's immunologically competent cells. This follows from the fact that splenectomy, prior to irradiation and inoculation of antigen, results in sensitization rather than unresponsiveness.

A-methopterin and X-irradiation have also been shown to act synergistically with crude cellular extracts of transplantation antigens in inducing tolerance in adult mice. Medawar found that the MST of C3H skin grafts on CBA animals which were exposed to 450 r and, 24 hours later, to 200 units* of a crude semisoluble extract prepared from C3H lymphoid tissue was more than 150 days, whereas their MST's on animals which had received irradiation or antigen alone were 57 days and less than 20 days, respectively. More modest degrees of unresponsiveness occurred with the A ⟶ C3H H-2 incompatible strain combination. Here, the MST of A strain grafts on C3H animals receiving 450 r and 250 units of A strain antigen was only about 30 days, as opposed to 22 days on irradiated recipients. However, some preliminary but clear suggestive evidence was obtained that this MST could be prolonged by increasing the amount of antigen given. These studies indicate that current procedures for prolonging organ homograft survival by means of drugs may be rendered much more effective by concomitant inoculation of the host with appropriately administered extracts of donor cells, especially when thay are reduced to a highly potent and completely soluble preparation (see Chapter 4).

Theories of Tolerance

A variety of theories have been propounded to account for the phenomenon of immunological tolerance. Of these, the "stem-cell" theory was the first to gain support because it was able to account for many of the experimental results cited earlier. It postulated that mature, immunologically competent cells were constantly being produced from newly differentiated stem cells throughout life and that these, at some stage of their

---

* The matter extracted from 200-mg wet weight of lymphoid tissue.

maturation, could respond to antigens by becoming tolerant rather than immune. Exposure of adult animals to antigen resulted in sensitization of the mature immunologically competent cells on the one hand, and the induction of tolerance in their functionally immature progenitors on the other. The immunological reactivity of the host was the summation of these two processes. Obviously, an immune response would normally cancel any tolerance induced. But appropriate tactics of antigen administration could lead to a shift in the constitution of the mature lymphoid cell population from a sensitized to a tolerant one, either by the elimination of immunologically activated cells as a consequence of prolonged contact with antigen, or by rendering them specifically "paralyzed."

An alternative possibility, and one which seems more attractive in the light of more recent information, is that proposed by Michie and Howard. They maintain that the target of the tolerance-inducing stimulus is the immunologically competent cell, and not an immature precursor or stem cell. Thus the ease with which tolerance can be induced in neonatal mice, as opposed to adult recipients, merely reflects the fact that neonatal animals possess exceedingly small numbers of immunologically competent cells. A deficiency in the macrophage activity of these animals may also be a contributing factor since phagocytosis and "processing" of antigen by macrophages appears to be an early step in the production of some immune responses. Indeed, there is evidence that, in the absence of macrophages, or if these cells can be bypassed, the direct action of antigen on lymphoid cells results in tolerance rather than immunity. The superior results obtained in inducing tolerance with intravenous inoculations, as opposed to other routes of antigen administration, may also be related to this fact.

In addition to the methods already mentioned for inducing tolerance of skin homografts in mature animals, specific unresponsiveness can sometimes be induced in mice simply by exposure to homografts of ovary, testis, or neonatal skin; in hamsters by prior exposure to cheek pouch or neonatal skin; and in chickens by previous conditioning with ovarian or testicular grafts (see Chapter 6). The capacity of these tissues to induce unresponsiveness in many instances is incomplete and usually applies only to situations where relatively minor histoincompatibilities prevail. For example, in contrast to the uniform rejection of adult male skin isografts by C57BL females, neonatal male skin isografts are frequently accepted. Moreover, 50% of all females which accept a neonatal male skin isograft for fifty days accept a subsequent adult male skin isograft as well. Similar results can also be obtained with ovarian grafts implanted subcutaneously, or with ovarian or testicular fragments transplanted to the spleen of H-1 or H-3 incompatible recipients. In other words, after these grafts have been in residence for fifty days, skin homografts of the same genotype are usually permanently accepted. Pregnancies resulting from matings between genetically unrelated mice may also result in tolerance (see Chapter 12).

The means by which tolerance can be induced in adult hosts, following exposure to appropriate kinds of solid tissue or cellular homografts, or through multiparity, as well as its relationship to the more orthodox methods of rendering animals unresponsive, remains to be determined. However, inasmuch as these procedures for inducing tolerance in adult subjects seem unlikely to be dependent upon the employment of large amounts of antigen, it raises the possibility that chronic exposure to small doses of antigen, presented in appropriate form, can also specifically paralyze the host. These findings certainly emphasize that tactics of antigen administration are important in determining whether tolerance or immunity will result. They also bring to mind the intriguing findings of experiments recently described by Mitchison on the dose of a soluble heterologous protein antigen, bovine serum albumin (BSA), required for the production of tolerance in mice.

Mitchison inoculated adult mice with various doses of BSA three times a week for varying periods of time. The animals were then challenged with BSA in adjuvant to determine whether they had become tolerant or immune. Two zones of tolerance could be defined. The first required high cumulative doses of antigen (>5 mg), appeared late in the treatment period, and was accompanied by an initial period of sensitization. The second required much lower doses of antigen (10 to 40 μg), was more immediate in its onset, and apparently did not involve a coincident state of immunity. On the other hand, cumulative doses of antigen which were intermediate produced immunity. Mitchison has interpreted these findings to indicate that virgin, immunologically competent cells confronted with antigen have two directions of response open to them—toward tolerance or toward immunity. The direction taken depends on the nature and concentration of antigen and on the extent to which macrophages process the antigen. Subimmunizing doses of antigen paralyze or render most of the appropriate immunologically competent cells tolerant, while a few become "primed" and, with more antigen, the sequence of events culminating in the production of immunity is completed. Once primed by antigen, competent cells are hyperactive, possess a higher paralysis-threshold, and therefore cannot be paralyzed by antigen except at much higher doses. Confronted by high concentrations of antigen, most cells become paralyzed and some become immunized. If the antigen administration is continued, even the sensitized cells become paralyzed (or are eliminated) and antibody production decreases. Immunizing doses of antigen, not high enough to paralyze sensitized cells, result in the proliferation of immunologically competent cells and the consequent production of high levels of antibody.

Tolerance as an Important Development Process

So far, the phenomenon of tolerance has been considered only as it applied to antigens of extraneous origin which accidentally gain access to developing embryos or are introduced experimentally into very young or adult animals. However, as Burnet and Fenner were well aware, some explanation is required as to why the cells which mediate an animal's immunological responses do not normally react against some of the differentiated constituents of its own body, i.e., why *autoantibodies* are not formed. Paul Ehrlich appreciated this philosophical problem more than half a century ago when he formulated his law of "Horror autotoxicus," which implies that autoantibodies are incompatible with normal life.

Since cells of the lymphoid tissue system either possess (are genetically tolerant of) or, from an early stage of development, are exposed to, and therefore acquire tolerance of all of the antigens responsible for transplantation immunity, this problem does not involve these antigens. However, many of the cells and tissues of the body do develop specialized substances as they differentiate, which they obviously do not share in common with the antibody-producing cells, and which might therefore appear foreign or antigenic to the latter. The most plausible reason why an individual's reticulo-endothelial system does not react against these substances is that it becomes exposed to them at a fairly early stage of development, and so becomes tolerant of them.

It follows from this argument that any specialized tissue constituent which is not produced until after the functional maturation of an animal's immunological response mechanism should be at least potentially autoantigenic. Likewise, specialized tissue constituents that develop in what is effectively a physiological quarantine, so that they do not gain access to the host's reticuloendothelial system, should also be potential autoantigens. Examples of both categories of substances are known. Spermatozoa develop relatively late in life and, if appropriately administered, will elicit the formation of autoantibodies against some of their distinctive components. Of course, they never get an opportunity to do this under normal conditions. The lens of the eye, on the other hand, develops at a fairly early stage of development but is encapsulated and physiologically isolated from the reticulo-endothelial system—it has no vascular supply. It is scarcely surprising, therefore, that it possesses protein ingredients which are potentially autoantigenic. The protein, thyroglobulin, appears to belong to this category, too. It develops in what appears to be an effective physiological quarantine—the follicles of the thyroid gland—from which it does not normally escape into the circulation. Consequently, this substance remains potentially autoantigenic. Witebsky and his associates established this fact when they demonstrated the autoantigenicity of thyroglobulin when it was administered to experimental animals under appropriate conditions. Presumably as a consequence of leakage or a lesion, it appears that thyroglobulin does escape just occasionally in man. When this happens, the regional or draining lymph nodes are stimulated to elaborate antibodies which circulate in the blood stream, and there is an infiltration of the thyroid gland itself with cells believed to be capable of forming antibodies. The result is a progressive thyroiditis and impairment of glandular function.

Of course, just as tolerance can be induced experimentally in adult life by appropriate amounts and tactics of exogenous antigen administration, it probably can also be induced in essentially similar ways to potentially antigenic substances which may develop for pathological or other reasons during the course of one's lifetime. This may explain, for example, the apparent nonreactivity of adult hosts against autochthonous tumors which are known to possess tumor-specific antigens.

The most convincing evidence available that non-reactivity to "self" components develops as an adaptive process during early life stems from an ingenious series of experiments carried out by Edward Triplett. This investigator extirpated the hypophyses of tree frog embryos at a stage in development before the gland had differentiated (i.e., begun to produce adult type proteins) but after it had been determined (possessed the ability to self-differentiate). These hypophyses were implanted temporarily in the dermis of other immature animals. When the animals from which these organs were removed had attained immunologic maturity, the explanted hypophyses which, by this time, had also differentiated were restored to them as dermal implants. In a significant proportion of cases, they were rejected. To exclude the possibility that their specificity had changed as a result of their having developed in a secondary host and incorporated some of its cells, in another series of experiments, Triplett removed only part of the hypophysis, cultivated it as before, and again returned it to the original donor. In these cases the grafts were always permanently accepted.

REFERENCES

Billingham, R. E., G. H. Lampkin, P. B. Medawar, and H. L. Williams. 1952. Tolerance to homografts, twin diagnosis, and the freemartin condition in cattle. Heredity 6:201–212.

Billingham, R. E., L. Brent, and P. B. Medawar. 1956. Quantitative studies on tissue transplantation immunity. III. Actively acquired tolerance. Roy. Soc. (London), Philos. Trans., B. 239:375–414.

Billingham, R. E., and W. K. Silvers, 1971. The immunobiology of tissue transplantation. *In* M. Samter, H. L. Alexander, D. W. Talmage, B. Rose, W. B. Sherman, and J. H. Vaughan [ed.] Immunological diseases, 2nd ed. Little, Brown and Co., Boston.

DeWeck, A. L., and J. R. Frey. 1966. Immunotolerance to simple chemicals. Monographs in Allergy, 1. S. Karger, Basel and New York.

Dresser, D. W., and N. A. Mitchison. 1968. The mechanism of immunological paralysis. Advances in Immunol. 8:129–181.

Hraba, T. 1968. Mechanism and role of immunological tolerance. Monographs in Allergy, 3. S. Karger, Basel and New York.

Nossal, G. J. V. 1968. Immunologic tolerance, p. 643–654. *In* F. T. Rapaport and J. Dausset [ed.] Human transplantation. Grune and Stratton, New York.

Owen, R. D. 1945. Immunogenetic consequences of vascular anastomoses between bovine twins. Science 102:400–401.

Chapter 11

Graft-Versus-Host Reactions

In the conventional graft-to-host relationship with which we have so far been concerned, confrontation of an immunologically mature individual with a homograft normally results in the destruction of the entire alien cell population: the host, as it were, recovers from an "attack" of foreign cells in a manner analogous to its recovery from an infection with microorganisms. This chapter deals with reactions that arise when, as a result of certain definable circumstances usually, though not exclusively, experimentally contrived, the immunologic roles of graft and host are reversed: cellular elements within the grafts react against their *hosts,* often with dire consequences (see Fig. 11.1). These reactions have been intensively studied over the past thirteen years, principally because: (1) they have afforded invaluable tools for studying immunologically competent cells; (2) they provide spectacular and easily reproducible examples of the damage that misdirected or abnormal immunologic reactivities can cause; and (3) they are very rarely encountered clinically.

Graft-versus-host (GVH) reactions have an interesting history. They were first studied unwittingly by Dr. James B. Murphy at the Rockefeller Institute in 1916. He observed that inoculation of the chorioallantoic membranes of young chick embryos with fragments of spleen, or certain other tissues, from adult chickens caused a striking enlargement of the *host's* spleen and the development of whitish nodules on the membranes, in the spleen and elsewhere. He noted that these nodules frequently had necrotic centers and that they comprised accumulations of leukocytes of various types. Unable to obtain evidence of a bacterial etiology, Murphy attributed the phenomenon to stimulation of the host's spleen and subsequent proliferation of its leucocytes in various sites. Subsequently, these observations were confirmed by Dr. Vera Danchakoff and others, who showed that similar grafts from embryonic donors, or very small grafts from adult donors, were ineffective.

In 1949 Drs. Brandley, Thorp, and Prickett found that what they presciently called the "embryo *disease*" was also provoked by inoculation

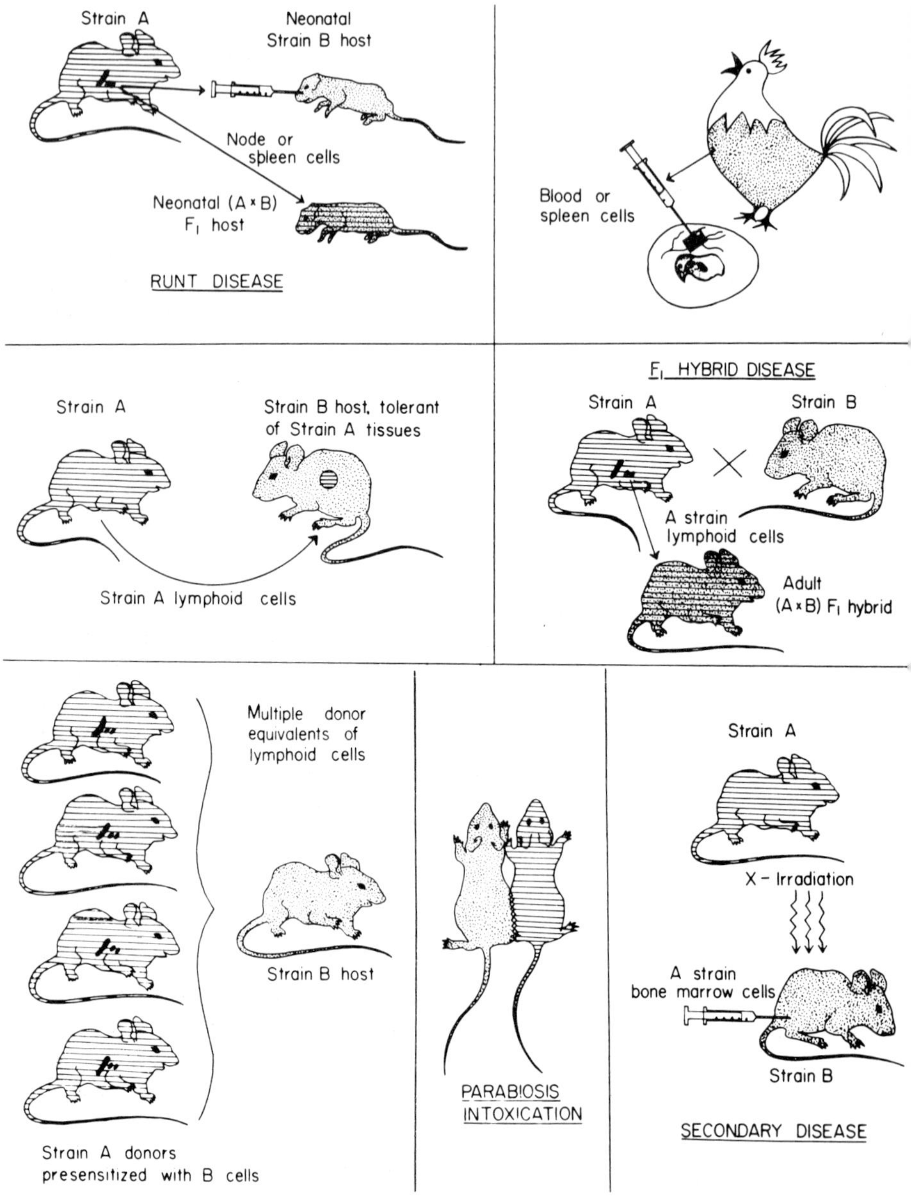

Fig. 11.1. A variety of different experimental situations in which homologous or graft-versus-host disease syndromes can develop.

of chick embryos with blood from normal, homologous adult donors, though this significant observation attracted little attention at the time.

The striking enlargement of an embryo's spleen, resulting from its inoculation with splenic tissue from an *adult* donor, was particularly intriguing to experimental embryologists, some of whom ascribed it to "organ-specific growth stimulation." For want of a more plausible alternative, this explanation enjoyed wide acceptance for a number of years.

The novel idea that grafts might, under certain circumstances, be capable of reacting against their hosts was first expressed, independently, in 1953 by Dr. W. J. Dempster in London and by Dr. Morten Simonsen in Copenhagen. While investigating the fate of renal homografts in dogs, these investigators were impressed by the very early appearance—within three to four days of grafting—of abundant pyroninophilic cells of the plasma cell family in the renal cortex. These cells had been shown by others to be involved in antibody formation when present in lymphoid tissue. On this basis both Dempster and Simonsen suggested that these cells were of local *graft* origin and that they were probably immunologically competent cells engaged in the process of responding immunologically against the alien transplantation antigens of the host perfusing the vascular bed of the grafted kidney. As we shall see, subsequent evidence that peripheral blood contains immunologically competent cells suggested an alternative explanation. In fact, it was later shown by other investigators that the plasma cells which excited Dempster and Simonsen were of host origin.

In 1955 Billingham, Brent, and Medawar unwittingly encountered the embryo disease when, trying to induce tolerance of skin homografts in chickens by intravenous injection of ten- to eleven-day-old White Leghorn embryos with blood from adult Rhode Island Red donors, they found that 95% of the hosts died just before hatching. Since blood from embryonic donors was innocuous, adult blood failed to harm newly hatched hosts, and the inoculation of chick embryos with adult duck blood was also harmless, these workers tentatively ascribed the mortality they'd encountered to some kind of "infective" organism present in the blood of most adult chickens.

From general principles, the conditions under which grafts might, in theory, be able to react against their hosts can easily be formulated:

1. The graft, whether cellular or solid tissue, must contain immunologically competent cells.
2. The host must possess transplantation antigens that are lacking in the graft donor, so that the grafted cells are stimulated antigenically.
3. The host must be incapable of mounting an effective reaction against the graft to the extent that the latter has some security of tenure.

In 1956, independent work at two centers established the validity of

GVH reactions as reproducible phenomena. At University College, London, Billingham and Brent were studying the induction of tolerance of skin homografts in newborn mice by injecting them with viable suspensions of 5 to 10 $\times$ 10^6 spleen cells from adult donors of different strains. Splenic cells were used because of the ease with which they could be prepared in a form suitable for intravenous injection—the optimal route for tolerance induction. With some donor/host strain combinations, such as CBA $\longrightarrow$ A, the postoperative mortality was relatively low and most of the survivors proved to be highly tolerant of CBA skin grafts. However, on dissection, many apparently normal, tolerant animals displayed severe involution of some of their lymph nodes and occasionally of their spleens. With other donor/host combinations, notably C57 $\longrightarrow$ A, the consequences of injecting adult splenic cells into newborn hosts were much more dramatic. The subjects soon stopped growing, frequently suffered from diarrhea, and invariably became emaciated. Most affected animals died of an acute disease within a few days of the onset of symptoms, but a small proportion lingered on for a month or two as sick, stunted runts with sparse fur, a hunched posture, and a peculiar mincing gait. A very small number eventually recovered.

This syndrome was referred to as "runt disease" on a purely descriptive basis. All the available evidence favored the hypothesis that it was due to graft-versus-host reactivity. As examples: (1) the severity and incidence of the disease was greatest when donor and recipient were most disparate genetically, and it failed to develop when they were closely related, as in the case of the H-2 compatible strains CBA and C3H; (2) its severity was usually heightened and its onset accelerated if the offending cell inoculum was derived from specifically *presensitized* donors, analogous to the second-set phenomenon; finally, and most telling, (3) the disease did not develop if lymphoid cells from F_1 hybrid donors were injected into newborn hosts of either parental strain.

Also in 1956, Simonsen was carrying out experiments specifically designed to produce GVH reactions. He found that injection of eighteen day-old chick embryos or newly hatched chicks with spleen cells, whole blood, or peripheral blood leucocytes from unrelated adult donors usually caused prompt and often striking enlargement of the host's spleen and liver, accompanied by acute hemolytic anemia and a positive Coombs' reaction. The disease was normally fatal in the case of embryonic hosts. Simonsen also discovered that neonatal mice, inoculated at birth with spleen cells from homologous adult donors, develop splenomegally within about ten days.

Subsequently, runt disease, or essentially similar syndromes in adult individuals, were procured in many species including mice, rats, hamsters, rabbits, guinea pigs, monkeys, and man.

General Considerations of Runt Disease

Genetic Requirements

Extensive studies (described later) on runt disease and other manifestations of GVH reactivity, both systemic and local, have shown that they are much more exacting in their genetic requirements than are conventional host-versus-graft reactions. When the putative attacking cells are derived from unsensitized donors, an essential prerequisite is that the host *must* confront the graft with alien transplantation antigens determined by the major H locus for the species concerned. For example, with mouse strains CBA and C3H which, though alike at the H-2 locus, differ at many other histocompatibility loci and reject each other's skin grafts within about twelve to fourteen days, runt disease cannot be incited by lymphoid cell inocula, even at high dosage levels. A similar situation exists with the Ag-B locus compatible Lewis and Fischer rat strains, in which the MST's of skin homografts are short (Lewis ⟶ Fischer, 11.6 ± 0.3 days; Fischer ⟶ Lewis, 7.6 ± 0.4 days). Indeed, the capacity of lymphoid cellular inocula from an unsensitized adult donor of one strain to cause runt disease, or its equivalents, in hosts of another strain, affords a valid indication of the existence of a difference at the major H locus for the species concerned. However, even when compatibility prevails at major loci, GVH reactivity is frequently demonstrable if the donor of the cellular inoculum has been *presensitized* against the recipient's tissue antigens.

The Inciting Cellular Inoculum

The *dosage* of the cellular inoculum from spleen or lymph nodes is an important factor in determining whether the disease will develop and also whether recovery is possible. However, for any given strain combination and with cells from the same source, over a wide dosage range, both the time of onset of symptoms and the life-expectancy of affected subjects are remarkably constant.

The capacity of cells from a given tissue source to cause the disease is related to the proportion of lymphocytes it contains: bone marrow is relatively harmless; spleen, peripheral leucocytes (predominantly lymphocytes in rodents), lymph node cells, and thoracic duct cells represent inocula of increasing potency. Lymphoid cells from fetal or neonatal donors are harmless, as might be expected on the grounds of immaturity. Indeed, such cells probably become tolerant of their host's antigens. Thymocytes from adult donors are usually inocuous, even at high dosage levels—an important, early observation that indicated the existence of a profound biological difference between thymus lymphocytes and those obtained from lymph nodes (see Chapter 9).

The inability to cause runt disease on the part of inocula comprising homogenized lymphoid cells or intact lymphoid cells killed by such moderate procedures as freezing and thawing, X-irradiation, or by viable cells of nonlymphoid types has been well documented. It is important because it sustains the thesis that GVH reactivity is causally responsible for the disease, rather than some kind of pathogenic organism(s) inadvertently transferred from adult carriers to susceptible infant hosts.

One of the most important early contributions of studies on GVH reactions to immunology in general was the demonstration that normal mammalian or avian blood contains cells capable of causing runt disease, i.e., immunologically competent cells. Subsequent studies in rats revealed that cells obtained by cannulation of the thoracic duct—about 95% small and 5% large lymphocytes—are highly potent incitors of runt disease, and that it is the *small* lymphocyte moiety that is responsible. Since thoracic duct lymph returns recirculating pool lymphocytes from the efferent lymphatic pathways to the blood stream, this indicated that the immunological competence of blood is a function of cells having the morphological characteristics of small lymphocytes. This was confirmed by Dr. Hildemann and his associates, who carefully fractionated mouse blood and established the capacity of its small lymphocytes to cause runting.

Although, in the chicken, early evidence incriminated the large lymphocyte of the blood as the cell type responsible for GVH disease, more critical studies have shown that here, too, the small lymphocyte is the causal agent.

Situations in Which Systemic Disease Develops as a Consequence of GVH Reactivity in Adult Hosts

Although runt disease is the prototype of and exemplifies graft-versus-host diseases in general, it is pertinent to survey the situations in which adult animals may develop what have been collectively described as homologous or transplantation diseases.

Studies on runt disease have revealed that, with increasing age of the infant host at the time of inoculation, its susceptibility to the disease falls off rapidly. This is attributable to the swift maturation of the host's immunological response machinery which, apart from rendering it increasingly refractory to becoming tolerant of the alien attacking cells, makes it progressively capable of reacting against and thus destroying the attacking cells before they can harm the host. However, even when donor and recipient are adult animals, there are situations in which GVH reactivity can cause overt homologous disease:

1. If adult mice of one strain are injected with very large numbers of lymphoid cells, e.g., several donor equivalents per host, from specifically presensitized donors, they may develop homologous disease, presumably as a consequence of being overwhelmed by the attacking effector cells.

2. What is sometimes referred to as "F_1 hybrid disease" occurs if normal parental strain lymphoid cells are inoculated into genetically tolerant F_1 hosts. Despite their inability to react against the attacking cellular inoculum, such animals require much higher dosages of cells per unit body weight than much younger hosts to incite the disease. Why this is so is unknown. Prior whole-body irradiation lessens the dosage requirement, probably by creating more *Lebensraum* in the host's lymphohematopoietic tissue system.

3. Adult animals, previously rendered immunologically tolerant of the transplantation antigens of a donor of a different strain, may develop homologous disease if inoculated with relatively large numbers of lymphoid cells from members of that strain.

4. *Parabiosis intoxication* is a lethal, wasting syndrome, sometimes encountered when adult mice or rats are united parabiotically with unrelated partners of their own species. The most favorable situation for analysis of this syndrome is obtained by parabiosing parental strain animals with their F_1 hybrids so that immunologic activity can take place in *one* direction only—against the genetically tolerant hybrid partner which becomes "intoxicated." The clinical picture in this particular homologous disease syndrome is complicated by the occurrence of a shunting of blood from the hybrid to the parental strain partner, leading to polycythemia and anemia, respectively. However, apart from these hemodynamic complications, there is no doubt that GVH-type reactivity, acting from within the victim, both initiates and makes an important contribution to the disease.

5. Secondary disease in radiation chimeras. Mice and certain other animals exposed to normally lethal dosages of ionizing irradiation may recover if given a transfusion of viable bone marrow cells from either isologous or homologous donors. By several means, it has been shown that this rehabilitation depends upon the grafted cells or their descendants becoming established in the depleted, anatomically appropriate sites in the host—its marrow and lymphoid organs—giving rise to a so-called *radiation chimera*. Whereas animals restored with isologous marrow usually enjoy a long life span, the survival of those rescued by means of hematopoietic tissue grafts of homologous origin is usually curtailed. Animals that have

made an apparently complete recovery from the primary effects of radiation develop a "secondary wasting disease," usually culminating in death within a month or two. In 1956 Dr. John Trentin of Baylor University postulated that this, too, is the outcome of GVH reactivity, and a wealth of evidence has since been presented that this is indeed the case. It is worth pointing out that, among the homologous disease (or GVH) syndromes, which are to some extent named in accordance with the context in which they are procured, secondary radiation disease is unique in the sense that the immunologic attack takes place in a host already damaged by irradiation. This complicates the picture. A similar consideration applies to so-called drug chimeras, in the production of which immunosuppressive drugs have been substituted for radiation, and which are liable to develop homologous disease.

The Demonstrable Lesions in Homologous Diseases

When it was first established that splenomegaly is a result of GVH reactivity, it was generally assumed that proliferation of donor cells, under antigenic stimulation by the host, was responsible for the initial enlargement of both spleen and nodes. This assumption received some support from findings that the lymphoid tissues of animals suffering from runt disease are chimeric. However, subsequent, more critical analyses using chromosomally or otherwise labeled donor lymphoid cells to initiate the syndrome have shown that in mice, rats, and chickens the initial phase of hypertrophy of host lymphoid organs is largely attributable to proliferation on a massive scale of the host's *own* cells. What provokes this massive, proliferative host-cell response is still open to conjecture. It clearly cannot be explained as the result of antigenic stimulation of the host by the foreign donor cells since it occurs in hybrid hosts as well as in those of inbred strains. Some authorities have regarded it as a "protective" mechanism provoked by the effects of an antecedent GVH reaction in which the incitants may be either the products of cell damage or destruction, or the liberated effectors of cellular immunity.

The relative paucity of demonstrable donor cells in the lymphoid organs of animals suffering from runt or F_1 disease may help to explain the difficulty of passaging these syndromes by transfer of lymphoid tissues, or cell suspensions prepared therefrom, to appropriate hosts. In most investigators' experience, a primary passage or transfer can usually be accomplished, though only rarely can a secondary passage be accomplished. Sublethal irradiation of the hosts facilitates passage experiments, presumably by providing Lebensraum for the passaged cells to proliferate and become established, so that the number of inoculated donor effector cells required to generate overt symptoms of disease is greatly reduced.

Careful studies by Dr. J. L. Gowans and his associates at Oxford, in which labeled thoracic duct small lymphocytes were injected from parental strain rats into F_1 hybrids and into lethally irradiated mice, provided confirmatory evidence that the cells responsible for inciting runt disease and its homologues do indeed "home" to the host's lymphoid tissues. Within twenty-four hours of inoculation, a proportion of the labeled cells transform into large pyroninophilic cells, presumably as a consequence of antigenic stimulation by host antigens. Other findings indicated that these cells then undergo rapid division to produce lymphocytes of progressively decreasing sizes. The similarity between these cytological events in the lymph nodes of animals undergoing GVH reactions and the events in the draining nodes of adult animals rejecting skin homografts in the conventional manner (see Chapter 8), reinforced the conclusion that a common underlying mechanism is involved.

Despite overwhelming evidence that GVH reactivity is basically responsible for the development of the various homologous diseases, it is remarkable how few tissues are affected and how trivially they are damaged. In no sense can the pathological lesions be described as impressive. If the subjects live long enough or fail to succumb to the disease, the initial striking phase of hypertrophy of spleen and nodes usually gives way to a state of chronic involution, generally held to be the outcome of cell destruction. There is a rapid disappearance of lymphoblasts and lymphocytes from the follicular areas of these organs and an abnormal proliferation of hemocytoblast-like cells and basiphilic reticulum cells. Hepatomegally is often an early feature of the disease, and lesions in the gastrointestinal tract are frequently demonstrable. The hematological findings are extremely variable from species to species and are difficult to interpret. There is usually anemia, associated with a positive antiglobulin test, and a drop in the various components of complement. There may also be leukopenia, a drop in the platelet count, and decreased cellularity in the bone marrow, but never evidence of cell destruction in this tissue.

Skin lesions of varying degrees of severity are frequently associated with all the variant forms of homologous disease in all species, including man and other primates. They are particularly striking in rats afflicted with runt disease and in hamsters suffering from F_1 disease. When present, they are almost pathognomonic. Usually there is erythema and edema associated with the presence of mast cells and mononuclear infiltration of the dermis. There may be alteration of the organization of the collagen fiber architecture of the skin and degenerative changes in epidermal cells with hyperkeratinization, presumably a consequence of a burst of mitotic activity, and a weakening of the dermo-epidermal junction, resulting in areas of separation or sloughing of the superficial epidermis. There may also be disappearance of skin appendages.

These skin lesions have attracted a considerable amount of interest and posed the important question of whether they are due to a *specific* immunologic attack on the part of infiltrating donor lymphoid cells, essentially a sort of homograft reaction, or whether they are nonspecific peripheral consequences of an immunologically procured derangement of the host's metabolism, or the presence of cell breakdown products in its blood.

Skin grafting experiments in rats appeared to have settled this question decisively in favor of the former possibility. Established grafts having the same genetic constitution as the affected hosts developed lesions, whereas skin grafts having the same genetic and antigenic makeup as the putative attacking cells were unaffected. However, this conclusion may not hold true for all species. Dr. Wayne Streilein has been studying the etiology of the severe lesions which may develop throughout the entire integument in hamsters suffering from acute F_1 disease. In affected animals, in which the entire superficial epidermis is easily separable from the dermis, the skin lesions are not immunologically specific. Established skin grafts from the strain which provided the attacking lymphoid cells are fully susceptible to the disease.

Indirect evidence is gradually accruing that infection may play an important though not necessarily decisive role in the pathogenesis of these diseases. The fact that the brunt of the immunological attack unquestionably falls upon the host's lymphoid organs suggests that their immunologic competence might be impaired, rendering the animals highly susceptible to infection. Studies on adult mice suffering from F_1 disease have afforded results in accord with this interpretation, the victim's response to particular pathogens usually being inversely related to the severity of the disease. Debilitation of the immunological response of animals suffering from homologous disease is evidenced by their tardy rejection of first-set homografts from third-party donors, by loss of preexisting sensitivity to homografts, and by impaired ability to react against Salmonella typhi H antigen or to T_2 phage. Inability to react against the latter is demonstrable even while the homologous disease is in its initial, subclinical stage.

One might have thought that some components of the lymphoid cellular inoculum responsible for inciting GVH disease would have conferred immunological protection upon the host by proxy. This seems not to be the case. Only when the cellular inoculum is provided by donors that have been immunized against a particular pathogen does it afford protection to its hosts.

Very pertinent to an understanding of the responses of homologous disease victims to bacteria is the fact that the proliferative phase of the disease is characterized by hyperphagocytosis. Dr. J. G. Howard and his colleagues have shown that nearly all the Kupfer cells present in the host's liver sinusoids (which are responsible for this activity) are of donor origin and that small lymphocytes present in the thoracic duct lymph can transform into this type of macrophage.

There is also a profound drop in the immunoglobulin and complement levels of affected mice in the acute phase of the disease. These deficiencies may be important in accounting for the mortality.

At present it is by no means proven that, for homologous disease to have a fatal outcome, the thriving of pathogen(s) in immunologic cripples is necessary. Indeed, the fact that runt disease develops in so-called germ-free mice suggests that the fulfillment of the disease may not be pathogen-dependent.

Local Graft-Versus-Host Reactions

Apart from the GVH reactivity which in some way or other causes the homologous diseases, it is possible to have localized GVH reactions following the inoculation of immunologically competent cells into certain sites. The classic example, already mentioned, is afforded by the white "pocks" that develop at sites of deposition of adult chicken splenic cells or peripheral leucocytes over the surface of the chorioallantoic membranes of homologous embryos.

Intrarenal GVH Reactions

If lymphoid cells from parental strain donors are injected beneath the renal capsules of appropriate adult Ag-B incompatible F_1 hybrid rats, a local invasive-destructive reaction occurs which can destroy up to 25% of the parenchyma of the affected organ (see Fig. 11.2). This apparently simple GVH system has been analyzed in detail by Dr. William Elkins. By employing cytologically "tagged" donor lymphocytes, he demonstrated that, after a latent period of two to three days, there is a period of at least five days of extensive proliferative activity on the part of the donor cells, giving rise to a rapidly dividing population of hemocytoblast-like cells. This proliferative activity on the part of the donor cells parallels the growth of the lesion, which subsequently regresses. These reactions are normally self-limiting and do not become systemic, though the regional or draining lymph nodes are frequently involved. In both its time course and its histopathology, this local GVH reaction is very similar to that which takes place in renal homografts undergoing acute rejection by normal

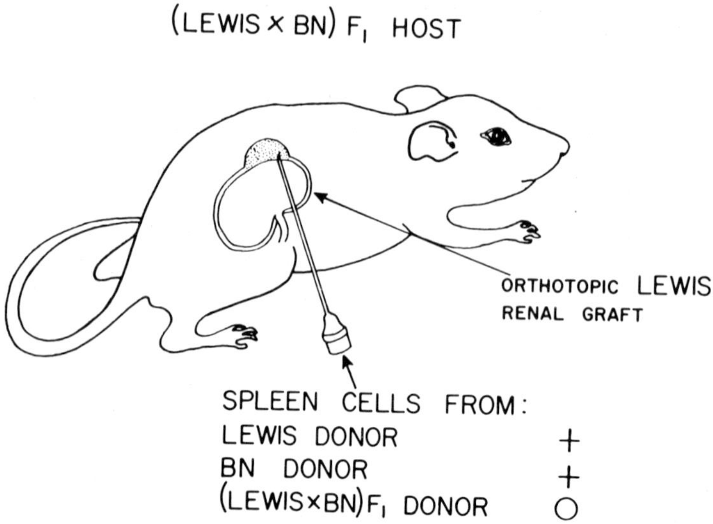

Fig. 11.2. The local graft-versus-host reaction system in the kidney employed by Elkins. A suspension of donor lymphoid cells is inoculated beneath the capsule of the host's kidney. Depending upon the genetic constitution of donor and host, an intense local cellular reaction culminates in loss of renal parenchyma. In the experiment illustrated, the (Lewis × BN) F_1 host has received a kidney graft from a Lewis strain donor. When splenic cells from either Lewis or BN donors were injected beneath the capsules of these organ grafts, local GVH reactions (+) developed.

hosts. This lends credence to the premise that the infiltrating mononuclear cells are engaged upon an attack against the renal parenchyma.

Elkins observed no increase in the tempo of the reaction nor its severity when cells from presensitized donors were employed. This is consistent with Simonsen's findings on GVH reactivity in chickens and suggests that, where major histoincompatibilities are involved, sensitization causes very little change in the proportion of reactive cells present. However, where only weak antigens are concerned, sensitization may cause a sixty- to seventy-fold increase in the proportion of these cells (see Chapter 8).

During their early developmental phase (up to the eighth day, post-inoculation), Elkins found that the local intrarenal GVH reactivity was transferable, by means of cell suspensions prepared from the lesions, to the kidneys of secondary F_1 recipients. This indicates persistence of the donor cell population and its capacity to continue effective GVH reactivity for at least seven days.

Subsequent analysis revealed that these local renal GVH reactions are not as simple as they first appeared to be. Prior irradiation of the host was found to inhibit their development to an extent related to the irradiation damage to the host's lymphoid tissue. This led Elkins to conclude that development of overt lesions in the host kidney depends upon a continuous reaction of specific reactive donor cells with a population of host mononuclear cells. Recently Elkins and Guttman have obtained confirmatory evidence for this premise. They have shown that a Lewis rat kidney still displays a typical local GVH reaction when, following its orthotopic transplantation into a (Lewis × BN) F_1 adult host, it is inoculated beneath its capsule with Lewis spleen cells. This reaction occurs even though the putative attacking cells and the kidney into which they are inoculated are of the *same* genetic constitution (Fig. 11.2). This important observation can have only one possible interpretation: donor lymphoid cells are stimulated antigenically by host, i.e., F_1, leucocytes passing through the vessels of the transplant, and the interaction of these two cell populations causes *nonspecific* damage to the renal parenchyma. This evidence is consistent with the postulated existence of a nonspecific cytotoxic effector(s) associated with the attacking cells. On the basis of these findings, Elkins raises the interesting possibility that passenger leukocytes in organ homografts may play an important role as immunogenic agents (see Chapter 8) and suggests that attempts to get rid of such cells might be a worthwhile endeavor. It is implicit in this line of reasoning that the indigenous cell population in an organ graft may be immunogenically feeble.

Intracutaneous GVH Reactions

If suspensions of lymphocytes from normal adult donors are injected into the skins of homologous guinea pigs, hamsters, sheep, men, and certain other species, they may incite local inflammatory reactions of delayed onset which are manifestations of reactivity on the part of donor immunologically competent cells against alien transplantation antigens of the host. As discussed in Chapter 2, the intensity of these normal lymphocyte transfer (NLT) reactions affords a measure of the antigenic disparity between donor and host. Of course, unless F_1 hybrid hosts are employed, the host normally reacts against the foreign cells deposited in its skin; thus, in its final stages, the reactivity observed is compounded by a conventional host-versus-graft reaction. If cells from presensitized donors are employed, the immune lymphocyte transfer (ILT) reactions develop sooner and are more intense.

In a study of both the normal and the immune lymphocyte transfer reactions in hamsters, Ramseier and Billingham found that prior whole-body irradiation of the host, which greatly depresses the peripheral leucocyte count, also greatly impairs the host's capacity to give these reactions. They also found that, if MHA strain hamsters which were tolerant of CB tissue antigens and chimeric with respect to CB cells in their lymphohematopoietic tissue system were injected intracutaneously with MHA anti-CB sensitized lymphocytes, ILT reactions developed. On the basis of these and other findings, they suggested that in all intracutaneous GVH reactions the antigenic stimulus against which the donor cells react in the host's skin is afforded not by the native cell population of this organ but by host *leucocytes* which percolate its vascular bed and, to some extent, traverse its parenchyma.

It is worth commenting that Brent and Medawar made use of these local GVH reactions in guinea pigs' skin to study the mode of action of various immunosuppressive agents (see Chapter 13).

Assay Procedures for Graft-Versus-Host Reactions

Although the capacity of cellular inocula to cause fatal runt disease affords a useful means of detecting immunologically competent cells, it is a rather insensitive test system complicated by the fact that certain pathogenic infections cause symptoms resembling those of runt disease. Various pathologic effects provide the basis of more reliable and more sensitive test systems.

Splenomegaly

Splenomegaly in infant mice and avian embryos is particularly favorable for quantitation. Simonsen has skillfully developed and employed this assay to elucidate a variety of fundamental problems in immunology, including analysis of the phenomena of sensitization and tolerogenesis. The simplest assay of splenomegaly entails comparison of the absolute spleen weights of test animals, which are usually killed eight to ten days after neonatal injection with adult lymphoid cells, with the spleen weights of uninjected controls of similar age and genotype. However, since the spleen weights of uninjected animals are positively correlated with their body weights, the relative spleen weight, i.e., the *ratio* of spleen weight to body weight, affords a useful measure of the enlargement of this organ caused by GVH reactivity.

One of the most useful measures of splenomegaly is the *spleen index,* calculated for each experimental animal by dividing its relative spleen weight by the mean of the relative spleen weights of control littermates. An index of 1.0 is indicative of no change in spleen weight, whereas an index of 2.0 represents a doubling of spleen weight. In a typical experiment, a standard number, e.g., 10^7, of parental strain spleen cells are injected intraperitoneally into some members of a litter of newborn F_1

hybrids. Eight to ten days later both the injected and uninjected control animals are killed and their body weights and spleen weights recorded.

Phagocytosis Assay

The phagocytosis assay is based upon the hyperphagocytic activity of the reticuloendothelial system associated with the proliferative phase of the GVH reaction in homologous diseases. It involves determination of the rate of clearance of colloidal carbon injected into the host's blood stream and is usually employed in adult F_1 hybrid mice injected with parental strain lymphoid cells.

Weight-Gain Assay

Developed by Russell, the weight-gain assay takes advantage of the fact that the weight of an infant mouse increases linearly over the first thirty days of its life. An abrupt cessation of weight gain affords an early indication of runt disease.

Chorioallantoic Membrane (CAM) Assay

The chorioallantoic membrane assay was studied by Sir Macfarlane Burnet and his associates in Australia. If a suspension of immunologically competent cells is distributed over the "dropped" chorioallantoic membrane of a chicken embryo, a number of white focal lesions or pocks develop within four to five days. These have been shown to be expressions of local reactions on the part of immunologically competent donor cells against the host's transplantation antigens. Appropriate analyses have shown that the activity of a single donor immunologically competent cell can produce one lesion. In fact, recent evidence indicates that here, too, the lesions are caused by interaction of donor cells with host leucocytes, rather than the normal cellular constituents of the membrane.

The Prevention and Treatment of Homologous Diseases

Studies on the prevention of GVH reactions and the associated homologous diseases are important not only for the light they shed on the pathogenesis of these conditions, but also because of the need to know how to treat them when they are encountered clinically.

In infant mice and rats, the development of runt disease can be prevented if the hosts are injected intravenously or intraperitoneally with lymphoid cells from normal, adult isologous donors. However, the timing of administration of the protective inoculum is very critical, especially in the rat; little protection is afforded if more than two days elapse between inoculation of the putatively harmful lymphoid cells and the therapeutic inoculum. If the donor of the isologous protective cells has been presensitized against the antigens of the attacking cells, then administration of the isologous cells as late as five days after the potentially harmful homologous cells may still exert a protective effect. The ability of both normal and sensitized isologous lymphoid cells to prevent a lethal GVH reaction is obviously due to their equipping the host with an effective machinery of immunologic response.

Since cells of the lymphoid series are particularly susceptible to the action of specific humoral isoantibodies in the presence of complement (Chapter 7), it is not surprising that, in both mice and rats, antisera are more effective therapeutically than even sensitized cells in protecting animals against runt disease. Indeed, in rats, daily injections of isoantiserum may totally reverse the course of the disease even when initiated as late as ten to thirteen days after inoculation of the attacking cells and at a time when the hosts already present overt symptoms of the disease. Heterologous antilymphocyte serum (see Chapter 13) is also an effective (though not as potent as isoantisera) protective agent.

The observation that delayed treatment of infant rats with isoantisera or ALS results in complete recovery of potentially doomed hosts provides telling evidence that the fatal outcome of runt disease is not caused by irreversible lesions inflicted at a very early stage.

The mortality that would otherwise result from administration of adult lymphoid cells to homologous hosts can be reduced by removal of the host's spleen a few hours after it has received the cells. This fact, in conjunction with the finding that splenectomy is ineffective if performed *before* the cells have been administered, suggests that the cells normally settle out in this organ after injection. Indeed, the observation that the splenectomy of adult F_1 hybrid mice as late as eight days after they've been inoculated with parental strain spleen cells reduces the mortality from homologous disease suggests that the spleen continues to act as a major seat of reactivity, or a source of reactive cells.

Various immunosuppressive drugs are also effective in preventing the development of homologous disease. For example, Amethopterin, which reduces the incidence of secondary disease in mouse radiation chimeras, has also been shown to be effective in protecting infant mice from developing fatal runt disease.

Finally, another means of avoiding the development of homologous disease entails pretreatment of the *donors* with immunosuppressive agents. ALS is relatively innocuous and highly effective in this respect (see Chapter 13).

Occurrence of Runt Disease in Human Infants

It is now generally accepted that a small-scale traffic in cells between mother and fetus is a common event in pregnancy (see Chapter 12). It is therefore possible that, if sufficient maternal small lymphocytes gain access to an imunogenetically appropriate fetus and are not themselves promptly rejected, runt disease might occur naturally in man. In 1965 Dr. Kadowaki and his associates reported on a male infant who developed symptoms suggestive of homologous disease within a few weeks of birth. Particularly significant was the observation that the baby's peripheral blood lymphocytes displayed XX/XY chimerism. The authors consider that GVH reactivity by cells of maternal origin may have been responsible for this fatal disease. Primary thymic arrest possibly contributed to the infant's nonreactivity to the alien cells.

There are several reports in the literature of infants with hereditary thymic dysplasia developing fulminating and fatal forms of GVH disease as a consequence of attempts to reconstitute their immunological function with bone marrow transplants. Fortunately it is now possible to avoid untoward incidents of this type by employing marrow cell grafts from carefully matched sibling donors.

The fairly recent practice of intrauterine transfusion of fetuses affected by Rh sensitization of their mother has also inadvertently resulted in some cases of runt disease. Further incidents of this type can be avoided if blood intended for transfusion to the fetus is rendered free of viable lymphocytes.

Several workers have considered the possibility of using very high doses of whole-body irradiation to treat leukemia and then giving bone marrow transplants to replace the patient's malignant myeloid tissue. Experiments in mice, in which isologous marrow grafts were used for rehabilitation, indicated the difficulty of applying this principle on account of the survival of some malignant cells and the consequent recurrence of malignancy. However, when homologous marrow was used to restore the irradiated subjects, the tendency for recurrence of leukemia was lessened, though the hosts usually died of secondary disease. It is believed that the GVH reaction afforded an additional line of attack against the tumor cells that survived the irradiation and possibly against viral agents involved in the etiology of the malignancy. Dr. Mathé and his colleagues in Paris have heroically been trying to apply this principle to the treatment of human leukemia. Although no complete cures have yet resulted, and the undesirable effects of secondary disease have had to be treated, some useful remissions have been encountered.

Homologous Disease and Malignant Disease

Several authorities have drawn attention to similarities existing between the hematological abnormalities associated with homologous diseases and those associated with systemic lupus and related disorders in man. Resemblances also exist between Hodgkins' disease and certain lymphomas on the one hand, and homologous diseases on the other. A possible basis for these similarities, put forward a few years ago, was the premise that, if some lymphoid cells suddenly lost the ability to produce an important transplantation antigen, they would theoretically be capable of reacting against the animal of which they were part, producing a disease that would be indistinguishable from homologous disease. This interesting concept remains totally devoid of supportive evidence.

In mice, it has been shown that GVH reactivity may cause, or at least facilitate, the development of malignant lymphomas. For example, Drs. Schwartz and Beldotti injected young adult (C57 $\times$ DBA/2) F_1 mice with C57 spleen cells, protecting them from homologous disease by administration of amethopterin. Fifty percent of the animals subsequently developed lymphomas of *host* genotype.

Dr. Roy Walford has shown that, with two closely related strains of mice differing only at the weak H-1 locus, neonatal inoculation of hosts of one strain with adult splenic cells from the other strain causes an increased incidence of lymphomas, though no overt runt disease develops. A possible interpretation of these interesting findings is that GVH reactivity causes activation of latent oncogenic viruses.

Other Syndromes Resembling Homologous Disease

Since runt disease was first described in the mouse, a number of wasting syndromes that simulate it fairly closely have been found to result from such diverse treatments as neonatal inoculation of mice with sterile bacterial vaccines, neonatal thymectomy (see Chapter 9), administration of cortisol acetate, and neonatal infection with certain viruses such as polyoma and LCM. Many of these "diseases" fail to develop if the treated infant mice are maintained under germ-free conditions, though they do develop soon after transfer of previously treated animals to a conventional environment. The fact that runt disease *does* develop in germ-free mice appears to differentiate it from these other syndromes.

Conclusion

Despite the attention that GVH reactions have received, we are still very ignorant about the pathogenesis of the diseases they cause. In some ways the offending cell inoculum is comparable to an invasion or infection by pathogenic microorganisms. Evidence is mounting that the essential interactions that lead to all forms of expression of GVH activity are those between donor immunologically competent cells and circulating mononuclear cells originating from the lymphohematopoietic tissues of the host. Several authorities have drawn attention to the similarity that exists between GVH reactions and mixed leucocyte interactions (Chapters 2 and 8), and further studies on the latter may well clarify our understanding of the former.

References

Billingham, R. E. 1968. The biology of graft-versus-host reactions, p. 21–78. *In* The Harvey lectures, Series 62. Academic Press, New York.

Van Bekkum, D. W., and M. J. de Vries. 1967. Radiation chimeras. Logos/ Academic Press, London and New York.

McBride, R. A. 1966. Graft-versus-host reaction in lymphoid proliferation. Canc. Res. 26:1135–1151.

Micklem, H. S., and J. F. Loutit. 1966. Tissue grafting and radiation. Academic Press, New York.

Silvers, W. K. and R. E. Billingham. 1969. Studies on the immunotherapy of runt disease in rats. J. Exp. Med. 129:647–661.

Simonson, M. 1962. Graft versus host reactions. Their natural history and applicability as tools of research. Progress in Allergy 6:349–467.

Chapter 12

Nature's Transplants: The Maternal-Fetal Relationship From the Viewpoint of Transplantation Biology

We tend to regard transplantation as an unnatural act perpetrated by surgeons and experimental biologists. However, there are a few circumstances in which transplantation of cells occurs naturally. For example, there is some evidence that, in hamsters, mosquitoes may be able to transmit a particular reticulum cell sarcoma from affected animals, in which malignant cells are present in the blood stream, to normal animals. Likewise, normal hamsters may occasionally develop this tumor as a result of biting affected cagemates. In this species, paucity of segregating transplantation antigens is probably responsible for the success of these natural cell transplants. In the dog a venereal tumor is known which appears to be due to the survival and proliferation of transmitted malignant cells, rather than to transformation of host cells by a virus.

However, by far the most important of Nature's transplants is the mammalian egg which, following fertilization, undergoes implantation and subsequently develops into an "organismic" graft of impressive proportions in the maternal uterus. In outbred populations every pregnancy represents a natural parabiotic union and mutual exposure of mother and fetus to each other's potentially foreign tissues and cells. This situation exists since the fetus inherits from its father a variable number of transplantation antigens that are foreign to the mother, and fails to inherit from the mother all of her transplantation antigens (Fig. 12.1). Consequently, ever since the principles of transplantation immunology were established, an explanation has been sought for the empirical fact that, unlike homografts transplanted to most sites in the body, naturally im-

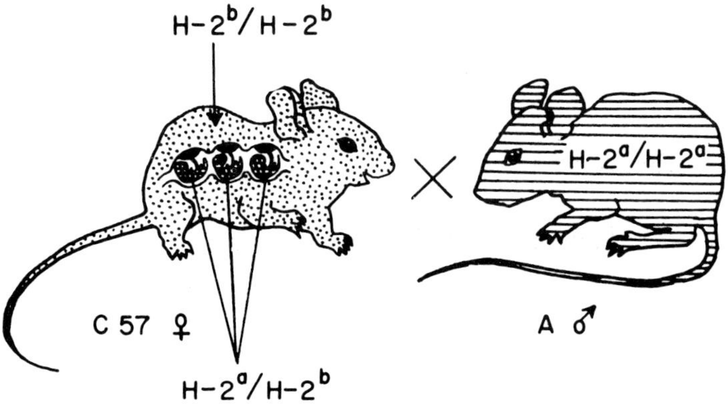

Fig. 12.1. This shows the potential immunogenicity of fetuses for their mothers to whose tissues they are intimately and parabiotically united. When a C57 female (H-2^b/H-2^b) is mated to an A strain male (H-2^a/H-2^a), all her fetuses will be heterozygous (H-2^a/H-2^b) and, consequently, will have an important transplantation antigen which is lacking in their mother. This will also apply to many other antigens determined by non-H-2 loci.

planted *embryos* in the uterus normally fail to incite an effective level of sensitization on the part of their mothers. Some idea of the magnitude of the homograft problem posed by pregnancy may be gained from the fact that females of many species, including mice and rats, can easily deliver several times their own weight of babies during their reproductive lifespan.

What might be construed as the earliest experimental study on the fetal homograft problem was performed in London by Walter Heape in 1890. He transferred two fertilized Angora rabbit eggs to the fallopian tube of a Belgian hare just mated with a buck of her own strain. In due course, the cuckolded mother gave birth to a litter of six baby rabbits—two of these were Angoras and four were Belgian hares (Fig. 12.2). In this experiment, the mother made no genetic contribution whatsoever to her Angora progeny; therefore, during their life in utero, their immunogenetic relationship to their "host" was similar to that which exists when homografts are exchanged between unrelated individuals. Subsequent work has shown that normal offspring will develop from transferred zygotes in other species, including mice, cattle, and sheep, with no overt immunological consequences.

With the exception of parthenogenesis, the only situation in which a fetus cannot confront its mother with any foreign antigens is when its parents belong to the *same* inbred strain, in which case it receives similar genetic endowments from both.

Not only are fetuses incapable of eliciting effective levels of sensitivity from their mothers, but they are also totally resistant to, and thus able

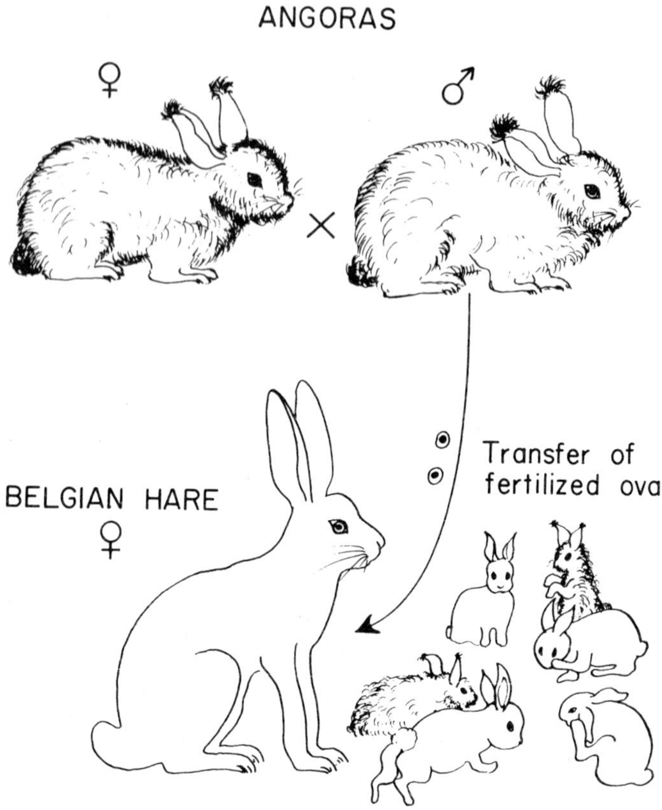

Fig. 12.2. Heape's foster pregnancy experiment. Two Angora rabbits were mated and two of the fertilized eggs transferred to the fallopian tube of a Belgian hare that had just previously been mated to a buck of her own breed. Subsequently, this animal gave birth to a litter of six young—four Belgian hares and two Angoras.

to override with impunity, an extant state of specific resistance evoked experimentally in the mother. For example, in *heterospecific matings* (those in which the parents are genetically disparate), preimmunization of the female against the alien tissue antigens of her consort fails to prejudice either the implantation or the normal development of zygotes. An experiment performed by Dr. Jonathan Lanman and his associates at Downstate Medical College, New York, demonstrated this in a particularly forceful manner. They were unable to impair the success of foster pregnancies in rabbits by prior *hyperimmunization* of the surrogate mothers, by skin grafting, against the tissue antigens of *both* parents of subsequently transferred blastocysts.

Hypotheses That May Explain the Anomalous Survival of the Fetus Quâ Homograft

Various hypotheses, which have been advanced to account for this virtually unqualified success of fetuses as homografts, will now be considered in relation to experimental evidence that bears upon them.

Complete Separation of the Maternal and Fetal Circulations is an Important Contributory Factor

All students of the problem have long been agreed that the complete separation of maternal and fetal blood circulations probably represents the most important protective factor. Circumstantial evidence sustaining this premise includes the fact that mammalian blood includes immunologically competent cells in its leucocyte moiety, capable of causing homologous or transplantation disease if they gained access to the fetus. Likewise, parabiosis of genetically disparate adult animals frequently results in an immunologically procured, normally fatal syndrome known as *parabiosis intoxication* (see Chapter 11). However, the vascular autonomy of the fetus per se is clearly unable to explain the inviolability of the fetus, since fetal and maternal tissues are intimately juxtaposed over a relatively large surface area in the placenta.

The Fetus is Antigenically Immature

The very plausible idea that the mother tolerates the growth of her embryos simply because the latter do not develop their isoantigenic individuality until relatively late in ontogeny was put forward by Dr. C. C. Little in 1924. However, so far as the fetus per se is concerned (we shall deal with fetal components of the placenta later), this explanation became untenable with the demonstration that transplantation antigens appear very early in embryonic life (see Chapter 4).

As for the extraembryonic tissues of embryos, their antigenicity was initially demonstrated by rather crude tests in which either intact or dissociated placental tissue from F_1 hybrid mouse fetuses, injected into normal mice of the maternal strain, induced immunity against subsequent skin grafts of paternal origin. However, such experiments failed to identify the antigenically effective components, which may well have been contaminating fetal leucocytes. Evidence that placental tissue homografts undergo accelerated destruction when transplanted to *presensitized* maternal strain hosts is more important since it establishes the vulnerability of at least some fixed components of this organ to transplantation immunity.

The Immunologic Reactivity of the Mother is Weakened During Pregnancy

There is some evidence, admittedly of a somewhat equivocal nature, that decreased resistance to certain infections is an accompaniment of pregnancy in man. During pregnancy there is increased production of adrenocortical hormones, some of which (especially cortisone) are known to impair the development of sensitivity to homografts as well as to other types of antigen. On this basis Medawar suggested that the immunologic capacity of the mother might undergo some kind of physiologic change that would protect the fetus against the risk of immunizing its mother. Support for this hypothesis was furnished by Drs. Heslop, Krohn, and Sparrow, who found that skin homografts transplanted to rabbits that were about three weeks pregnant (the gestation period in this species is thirty-two days) lived almost twice as long as grafts transplanted sooner or later in pregnancy or grafts transplanted to nonpregnant animals. This observation was tentatively ascribed to the enhanced steroid secretion during the latter part of pregnancy. However, neither pregnancy nor treatment with steroid hormones significantly weakens the level of a *preexisting* sensitivity to homografts in rabbits. Furthermore, neither in mice nor in cattle (gestation period about 280 days) does pregnancy affect a female's reactivity to skin homografts. Thus, at best, the increases in corticosteroid production associated with pregnancy, to which both placenta and fetus probably contribute, can only afford a weak ancillary mechanism for preventing maternal isoimmunization during pregnancy in a few species.

The Uterus is an Immunologically Privileged Site

As we saw in Chapter 5, there are certain privileged sites in the body in which grafts of alien origin may acquire a blood supply and yet thrive for a long time, apparently exempt from the rejection process.

However, various lines of circumstantial evidence make it difficult to believe that any kind of privileged status of the uterine milieu is responsible for the success of fetuses as homografts. In man, for example, ectopic pregnancies may occur in which *nonuterine* tissues or organs such as the fallopian tubes, the pelvic ileum, the rectum, and lateral and posterior aspects of the peritoneum in the pelvis form the implantation sites of the blastocyst and, subsequently, the site of attachment of the embryo's placenta.

Attachment at these aberrant sites does not necessarily prejudice normal development for a considerable period and, occasionally, to term. When fetuses do die under these circumstances, there have been no indications that homograft reactivity on the part of the mother is responsible.

In experimental animals, blastocysts caused to become attached to the mesenteries, or implanted beneath the renal or splenic capsules of genetically incompatible hosts, still develop into normal embryos.

Highly suggestive direct evidence that the uterus does not possess distinctive immunologic properties which make it a favorable attachment site for alien zygotes has been furnished by grafting experiments in which homografts of malignant or normal tissues have been caused to become established on the uterine wall. Dr. Michael Schlesinger found that tumor homografts were rejected in a perfectly orthodox manner after a transient period of growth, following transplantation to the uterine horns of rats and mice. A preexisting state of immunity was also fully expressed in this site.

One criticism leveled at the validity of this evidence was that the tumor homografts in utero may outgrow the limits of the physiological uterus, their destruction being due to penetration of *nonuterine* tissue. However, the fact that test homografts of a normal, noninvasive tissue, furnished by parathyroid grafts, are also destroyed in the uterus minimized this possibility, though it didn't refute it.

Dr. D. R. S. Kirby has suggested that the decidual reaction to a conceptus may in some way quarantine the embryo in an immunological sense. However, Drs. Beer and Billingham have recently shown that small, free-skin homografts grafted to the intact endometrial surface still incite and succumb to a typical homograft reaction even though they stimulate a decidual response.

In conclusion, therefore, with one qualification to be referred to later (see page 177), it is hard to ascribe the success of the fetus qua homograft to peculiar properties of the uterus.

A Physiological Barrier Exists Between Mother and Fetus

The most striking quality of the fetal homograft is its apparent invulnerability to a state of specific sensitivity in the mother directed against its own alien tissue antigens. This resistant property is expressed very dramatically in species whose placental structure is such (hemochorial placentae) that maternal blood, which bears the cellular effectors of transplantation immunity, is continuously in contact with a large aggregate area of trophoblast cells of the fetus (Fig. 12.3). In man, estimates of the aggregate

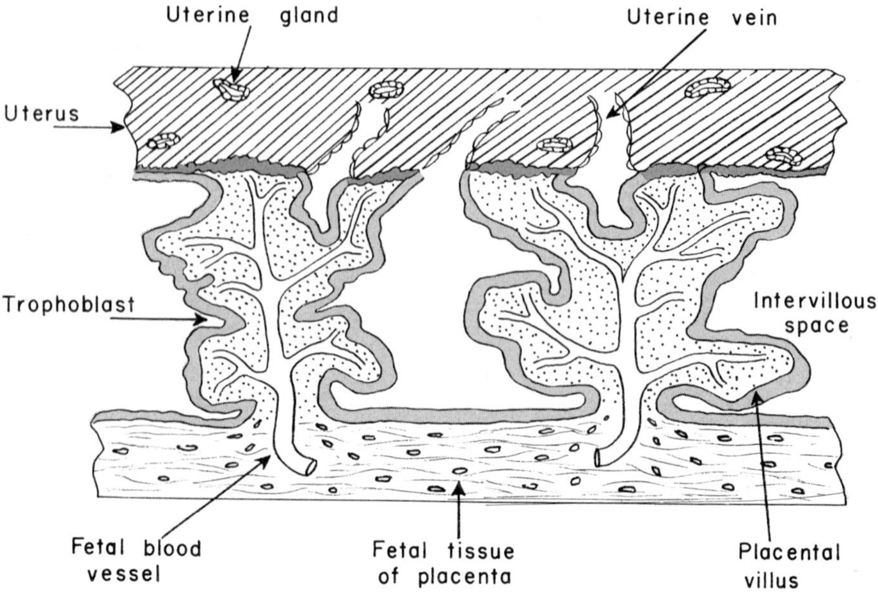

Fig. 12.3. This illustrates the extremely intimate relationship between maternal and fetal tissues in the human placenta. The trophoblast (light gray in drawing) forms an unbroken "frontier layer" of fetal tissue which is in contact with maternal uterine tissue, or blood (in the intervillous spaces). Note that the fetal blood vessels in the placental villi are separated from the maternal blood which bathes the villi by fetal connective tissue (dotted) surfaced by trophoblast.

area of trophoblast thus exposed range from ten to fifteen square meters.

Only one hypothesis is capable of accounting for the survival of fetuses in both normal and sensitized mothers: They are surrounded by some kind of anatomical barrier which: (1) normally prevents the mother from developing a state of transplantation immunity directed against the antigens of the fetus and (2) affords the fetus complete protection against high levels of immunity evoked in the mother experimentally. Simply because it represents a continuous, unbroken "frontier" component, attention has long been focused on the fetal trophoblast as holding the possible key to the riddle (Fig. 12.3). In hemochorial placentas found, for example, in mice, rabbits, guinea pigs, and man, only a very thin layer of trophoblast intervenes between many of the fetal capillaries and maternal blood in the intervillous spaces.

The idea that the placenta could function as a barrier if its trophoblastic cells were nonantigenic was put forward more than forty years ago by Dr. Ernest Witebsky and his associates on the basis of their observation that human placental villi are deficient in blood group antigens. Subsequent evidence, suggesting that normal trophblast may indeed possess interesting transplantation properties, was derived from studies on its malignant derivative, choriocarcinoma of gestational origin, a tumor encountered only in man. This highly invasive tumor, which metastasizes regularly via the veins of the mother and which may involve many organs, originates from the chorionic epithelium of the fetus. Despite the fact that these tumors are homografts, only rarely do they undergo regression in untreated subjects though, admittedly, their spontaneous regression rate is much higher than with all other types of human malignancy. This suggests that they are not always completely devoid of isoantigenic activity.

Recognition of the genetically alien nature of choriocarcinomas was followed by attempts at immunotherapy—by grafting affected women with skin or peripheral blood leucocytes from their husbands in the hope that the sensitivity evoked might exert an adverse effect on malignant cells. Unfortunately, almost without exception, this expedient was without beneficial effect. Indeed, some of the women behaved as if they had become specifically tolerant of their husband's skin, possibly because of prior chronic exposure to transplantation antigens of tumor cell origin, in some instances in the presence of anticancer (immunosuppressive) drugs such as methotrexate (see Chapter 10).

It is interesting to note that, in 1961, Drs. Hacket and Beech concluded that "choriocarcinoma is effectively nonantigenic because it exhibits the same mechanism or properties of physiologic nonantigenicity that exist in normal trophoblast." Although they have never been tested, it seems very probable that, unlike homografts of all other human tumors, those of choriocarcinoma would survive and thrive if transplanted to normal human subjects.

Carefully designed experiments in mice have provided strong support for the thesis that a normal trophoblast possesses properties that would enable it to function as an immunologic protective barrier between mother and fetus. Drs. Russell and Simmons analyzed the histocompatibility characteristics of mouse placental tissue at various stages of its development, studying grafts from F_1 hybrid embryos transplanted to adult hosts of the maternal strain. Under these conditions accidental inclusion of maternal cells in fetal tissue grafts cannot influence the host immunologically. When seven-day mouse conceptuses were separated into their trophoblastic and embryonic moieties and implanted beneath the renal capsules of maternal strain hosts presensitized against paternal strain tissue antigens, the embryonic grafts underwent prompt destruction. However, those of trophoblastic tissue displayed proliferative and invasive activity on the part of the giant cells, with the formation of typical blood spaces. These alien grafts survived just as well and for as long as similar grafts transplanted to genetically compatible hosts.

In 1959 Drs. Bardawil and Toy put forward the interesting suggestion that a local deposition of fibrinoid substance, known as the "layer of Nitabuch," which usually separates maternal from fetal tissue in the human placenta, may behave somewhat as an immunological no-man's-land, walling off the fetus from chemical interaction with its host. Subsequently Kirby and his associates, at the University of Oxford, presented various lines of evidence sustaining what is essentially this hypothesis. On the basis of histochemical and electron microscopical studies of mouse placentas, they reported that each trophoblast cell is surrounded by a layer of amorphous, electron-dense, fibrinoid material ranging in thickness from 0.1 to 2 μ. This material closely resembles the intracellular matrix of the connective tissue of the hamster's cheek pouch (Chapter 6), containing a mucoprotein rich in tryptophane with at least two nonsulphated acid mucopolysaccharides, probably hyaluronic and sialic acids. The amount of fibrinoid present was found to be related to the immunogenetic disparity between mother and her fetus. When there was no disparity, the trophoblastic cells were surrounded by less fibrinoid than when these cells were derived from F_1 hybrid embryos or from embryos resulting from transfer of blastocysts from one donor strain of mice to the uteri of pseudopregnant surrogate mothers of an unrelated strain. Since it appears that placental fibrinoid is secreted by trophoblast cells, the immunologic quarantining of the placenta resembles that of cartilage in the manner of its accomplishment (see Chapter 5).

At present there is insufficient evidence from other species to establish the general validity of Kirby's thesis that it is this peritrophoblastic layer of fibrinoid material that exempts this tissue from conventional homograft phenomena. However, the recent report by Drs. Currie, Van Doorninck, and Bagshawe that treatment of ectoplacental cone cells from 7½-day-old mouse embryos with neuraminidase unmasks the presence of transplantation antigens, enabling these cells to sensitize mice against subsequent skin homgrafts of the same genetic origin, lends considerable support to Kirby's thesis.

The Antigenic Status of Pretrophoblastic Egg Stages

The antigenic status of pretrophoblastic zygotes is a matter of considerable interest, and we shall now consider some of the evidence that bears upon it. If fertilized mouse ova, two and one-half days after conception, are placed beneath the renal capsules or into the spleens of isogenic hosts, they develop into tiny "tumors" of trophoblastic giant cells having a life span of about two weeks. No curtailment of this life span results if the hosts are genetically incompatible mice, nor do these grafts appear to elicit a detectable level of immunity. Furthermore, when transplanted to specifically presensitized females (by means of skin homografts), the behavior of these grafts remains unaltered, and they fail to elicit a local mononuclear cell response. It was subsequently found that, if homologous ova are transplanted beneath the renal capsules of male mice which have been specifically *hyperimmunized* against the tissue antigens of the zygote donor strain (by repeated skin grafting and inoculation of lymphoid cell suspensions), a significant proportion failed to develop into trophoblastic tissue. However, if trophoblastic tissue did develop, there was no evidence that its growth was impaired. Ectoplacental cones of seven-day embryos were found to be completely resistant to a state of hyperimmunity.

On the basis of findings such as these, Simmons and Russell suggested that transplantation antigens are present in pretrophoblastic egg stages and that trophoblast represents a differentiated or specialized form of embryonic cell characterized, among other things, by an inability to manufacture or express on its surface antigens that are displayed by its immediate precursors. The zona pellucida, which is impermeable to many proteins and to cells, probably affords immunologic protection to fertilized eggs prior to the formation of the trophoblastic barrier in a female which, for any reason, is hypersensitive with respect to her mate's tissue antigens.

Contrasting with the susceptibility of fertilized homologous eggs to transplantation immunity when grafted beneath the renal capsules of hyperimmunized hosts is the finding that they develop *normally* if transplanted orthotopically to the uterine horns of pseudopregnant hyperimmune females. To explain this difference, Kirby and his associates postulate that decidual cells, which do not develop in the kidney, may be responsible for the protection of the otherwise vulnerable embryos until they've developed their trophoblast-associated protective fibrinoid layer. In other words, decidual cells may confer an immunologically privileged status *locally* at implantation sites in the uterus. Another possibility worth considering is whether some kind of nonimmunological interaction between the implanting egg and the endometrium may result in the suppression of the synthesis of transplantation antigens.

In the light of these findings it is difficult to attribute infertility or early spontaneous abortions in women to sensitization against their husbands' transplantation antigens.

Drs. Hulka and Kirby and their respective associates have, independently, studied the influence of *repeatedly* grafting male mice of one isogenic strain with either ectoplacental cones, or blastocysts derived from mice of an unrelated donor strain. The grafts were implanted beneath the renal capsules or into the testes of the hosts. This procedure resulted in a progressive impairment of the capacity of later grafts to grow, and they incited progressively smaller hemorrhagic reactions. Even more striking was the observation that isogenic, i.e., genetically compatible, blastocysts also failed to develop normally when transplanted to mice which had previously received several sets of homologous blastocysts. Consistent with this observation was Kirby's finding that repeated exposure of C3H host strain mice to C3H blastocysts also resulted in progressive impairment of the ability of later grafts to thrive.

These observations suggest the existence of embryo-specific, probably trophoblast-specific, antigens whose existence had previously been postulated on the basis of indecisive serological studies.

It is worth recalling in this connection that Dr. Lewis Thomas tentatively suggested that degenerative changes occurring in normal placentas as gestation proceeds might be ascribed to sensitization of the mother to a special, organ-specific antigen, possibly one that appears rather late in the maturation of the placenta. Parturition might, therefore, represent an immunologic rejection, analogous to that of a homograft. Of course, as Thomas pointed out, one cannot implicate transplantation antigens in such a hypothesis, for then the hypothesis would fail to account for placental separation in isogenic strains.

The Influence of Antigenic Disparity and the Immunologic Status of the Mother on Placental Size

Although, as we've seen, neither the implantation nor the subsequent development of conceptuses in the uterus are affected by sensitivity directed against their foreign antigens, there is evidence, at least in the mouse, that growth of the placenta is influenced by both the genetic disparity between a mother and her embryos and by her immunologic status.

Dr. W. J. Billington found that mouse placentas tend to be larger when mother and fetus are genetically disparate than when they are alike —hybrid fetuses having larger placentas than fetuses whose parents were members of the same inbred strain. The possibility that this size differential simply reflected hybrid vigor was effectively ruled out by the observation that fertilized eggs from *homospecific matings* (i.e., those in which the parents are genetically similar), transferred to the uterus of a female of a *different* strain, produced larger placentas than they would have done if allowed to develop in their genetically similar mothers. Billington then showed that, when ectoplacental cones were transplanted to the testes, trophoblastic invasion of host tissue was greater where histoincompatibility prevailed than where graft and host were isogenic.

The influence of the immunologic status of the mothers on the placental size of their F_1 hybrid offspring has been studied by Dr. D. A. James. Apart from confirming that hybrid fetuses tend to have larger placentas than C57 fetuses in C57 mothers, he found that prior immunization of mothers to paternal strain antigens resulted in a significant increase in size of the placentas of F_1 hybrid offspring. Prior induction of tolerance in the mother with respect to paternal tissue antigens resulted in hybrid fetuses whose placentas were significantly *smaller* than those of similar fetuses carried by immunologically normal mothers. As James points out, if placental size is dependent upon the extent of trophoblastic invasion of the uterus, this invasion must be affected by the immunologic status of the mother in such a way that it is more extensive in immune and less extensive in tolerant than in normal mothers. Before the general significance of these observations can be appraised, similar studies must be carried out on the placentas of other species.

Choricarcinoma and Compatibility at the HL-A Locus

As already mentioned, there are clinical observations which suggest that choriocarcinoma is not always devoid of isoantigenic activity. Furthermore, the high proportion of complete remissions now obtainable by means of various anticancer drugs is consistent with the concept that, in many patients, some degree of sensitivity toward their tumor does arise.

A question of some clinical significance under current investigation at several medical centers is whether the degree of histoincompatibility between this tumor of fetal origin and affected females influences the course of the disease. One might expect that, in instances where these tumors are highly compatible with their hosts, the course of the disease might be more severe than in cases where the tumor was less compatible. A group of Danish workers studying this possibility have obtained data which suggests that tumors originating from HL-A *incompatible* fetuses show a significant tendency to remain localized within the pelvic region, whereas HL-A compatible tumors tend to become generalized. Furthermore, there was a significant difference with respect to HL-A2 incompatibility between husband and wife, which suggests that incompatibility between the malignant graft and the mother, with respect to this particular HL-A specificity, protects her from generalization of the tumor, restricting it to the uterus.

Possible Significance of Histocompatibility Antigen Polymorphism in Pregnancy

It has been suggested that in mice immunogenetic dissimilarity between mother and offspring favors placental development, as does the presence of maternal sensitization to antigens present in the fetus. This may afford the basis of a natural selection mechanism, capable of maintaining balanced polymorphism with respect to the great diversity of transplantation antigens in mammals.

In both mice and rats, some backcross matings of F_1 hybrid males with parental strain females have yielded an R_2 population in which there were significantly fewer than the expected 50% of the offspring that were homozygous for a particular segregating transplantation antigen. On the other hand, no disturbance in expected ratios occurred among the offspring of heterozygous females mated with homozygous males. Hull has recently found that this "autoincompatibility effect" is significant only in later litters; thus, it resembles the interaction between mother and fetus that causes Rh hemolytic disease in man, and which also increases with parity.

In a substrain of Wistar rats with a history of seventy-two generations of brother-sister matings, Michie and Anderson found that 52% of intrastrain skin grafts were still being rejected very promptly. Analysis revealed that this state of affairs resulted from a strong selective effect associated with a histocompatibility gene. The results were explicable on the hypotheses that two alleles, g_1 and g_2, were segregating in the population and that the survival value of the heterozygous individuals was superior to that of either homozygote. Litter size data indicated that the selective elimination occurred *before* implantation of the fertilized eggs. Michie and Anderson raised the interesting possibility that selective fertilization may occur, g_1 sperm uniting preferentially with g_2 eggs, and vice versa.

Maternal-Fetal Exchange of Cells and Its Consequences

The normal placenta is not a perfect, cell-impermeable barrier. Some transplacental traffic in cells between mother and fetus must now be regarded as commonplace in man and probably in many other species too, and this probably commences very early in ontogeny. The most cogent evidence relates to the exchange of erythrocytes, but evidence is also accumulating that leucocytes are also exchanged. In man, estimates of the amount of fetal blood gaining access to the maternal circulation range from 0.1 to 3.0 ml, but this amount may, on some occasions, be greatly exceeded. Direct evidence that maternal cells, especially red cells, normally enter the fetus, based on studies of cord blood, is much less convincing. The fact must not be overlooked that there is a blood pressure difference between fetal and maternal circulations favoring passage of cells from fetus to mother. As we shall see, this may have some protective advantage.

In some mammals, notably chinchillas and hamsters, trophoblastic cells may actually invade maternal blood vessels. In man, cellular fragments of the syncitiotrophoblast frequently, if not invariably, gain access to the blood stream of pregnant women from the eighteenth week of gestation onward. There is no evidence that these "grafts" of fetal origin ever proliferate or have any overt immunological effect. Indeed, they seem to undergo rapid enzymic dissolution.

Influence of Passage of Fetal Cells into the Mother

So far no convincing evidence has been produced that even *repeated* heterospecific pregnancies lead to the development of transplantation immunity directed against alien paternal strain antigens. However, such pregnancies can certainly lead to the formation of humoral isoantibodies in mice and man (see Chapter 2), probably as a result of small placental "bleeds."

With some strain combinations of mice in which only non-H-2 histoincompatibilities are involved, repeated heterospecific pregnancies do not lead to sensitization but may lead to exactly the opposite modality of response—a long-lasting specific *weakening* of the female's reactivity to test grafts of skin or tumor from the paternal strain. For example, the ability of BALB/c female mice to reject homografts from DBA/2 donors is progressively impaired as a consequence of repeated pregnancies by males of this strain, though with test skin grafts, abrogation of host reactivity never becomes complete. Where H-2 incompatibilities are involved, some weakening of host reactivity also results from heterospecific pregnancies, though a test homograft of tumor rather than skin is required to reveal it.

The histoincompatibility system in which the influence of parity exerts the most striking effect is that determined by the Y factor in C57BL/6 mice (see Chapter 3). Whereas practically every adult virgin female will reject a male skin isograft within about fifteen to fifty days (MST about twenty-seven days), irrespective of her age at the time of grafting, with increasing parity by males of their own strain, an increasing proportion of C57 females become totally incapable of rejecting male skin isografts. In our experience no female which has given birth to eight or more litters is able to reject male skin isografts. There is evidence that repeated insemination of naturally sterile or artificially sterilized C57 female mice also exerts a slight weakening effect on their subsequent reactivity to male skin isografts. This suggests that material, possibly spermatozoa, bearing the Y antigen and present in the semen, must somehow leave the genital tract of the female, gaining access to her tissues.

With the DBA/2-BALB/c combination there is evidence that the antigenic stimulus responsible for weakening the BALB/c female's capacity to react against grafts of DBA/2 skin originates from the conceptus. However, the means by which this antigenic material procures the specific weakening of response remains unknown. Since, in both mice and rats, repeated heterospecific pregnancies are known to result in the appearance of humoral antibodies in the mothers, the possibility that the phenomenon of immunological enhancement is at least in part involved cannot be excluded (see Chapter 7). However, low-dose tolerance affords an alternative, and not mutually exclusive, explanation (see Chapter 10).

Conceivably, more impressive results might be obtainable in animals with longer gestation periods. An important question, clinically, is whether repeated normal pregnancies weaken a woman's capacity to react against her husband's tissues.

Influence of Passage of Maternal Cells into the Fetus

If maternal cells, other than erythrocytes, gain access to and become incorporated in the fetus, the most obvious possibility is that, depending upon the degree of histoincompatibility and the number and type of maternal cells involved, some degree of tolerance of maternal tissue antigens will be induced. Various studies have been carried out to explore this possibility in various species. With outbred stocks of animals, these have simply entailed comparing the survival times of maternal and paternal homografts on their offspring. Where inbred strains of animals were available, experiments of a more sophisticated design have been employed.

Because of its long gestation period and hemochorial type of placenta, the guinea pig seemed to be a promising candidate for the occurrence of maternally induced tolerance. To evaluate this possibility, F_1 hybrids between two isogenic strains, #2 and #13, were reciprocally backcrossed to strain #13. This produced two similar genetically defined, but heterogeneous, populations of animals which differed only insofar as one group of animals had developed in an F_1 uterine milieu which had afforded them an opportunity to incorporate F_1 cells (bearing strain #2 antigens) prenatally. To test for any alteration of immunologic reactivity this may have caused, both groups of R_2 progeny were challenged, when they were thirty days old, with skin from strain #2 donors. Comparison of the distribution of survival times of the two groups of grafts revealed that they were very similar, indicating that maternally acquired tolerance must be a rare phenomenon in this species if it occurs at all. An experiment of similar design conducted upon mice of strains A and CBA yielded the same result.

Démant has shown that there is a slight but significant prolongation of survival of maternal, as compared with paternal, skin grafts transplanted to the newborn progeny of rabbits which are fairly closely related genetically. However, when test grafting was delayed by as little as three days after birth, the difference disappeared. When both parents belonged to different "lines" and the genetic disparity involved was greater, no prolongation of maternal graft survival was demonstrable. Indeed, in some instances, the findings indicated that some offspring may have been sensitized to maternal antigens during life in utero.

In collaboration with Dr. Joy Palm, we have employed a sensitive test for tolerance induction in rats, using the experimental design illustrated in Fig. 12.4. It is based on the observation that, whereas three-day-old Lewis rats reject skin grafts from adult BN donors as vigorously as do adult hosts, three-day Lewis rats inoculated at birth with as few as 1×10^6 BN marrow cells display some degree of tolerance of BN skin grafts. In our experiments, adult (BN × Lewis) F_1 hybrid females were given orthotopic Lewis ovarian grafts of which they were genetically tolerant. These animals were subsequently mated with Lewis males to produce offspring of Lewis genotype which, as a result of gestation in an F_1 maternal milieu and suckling by F_1

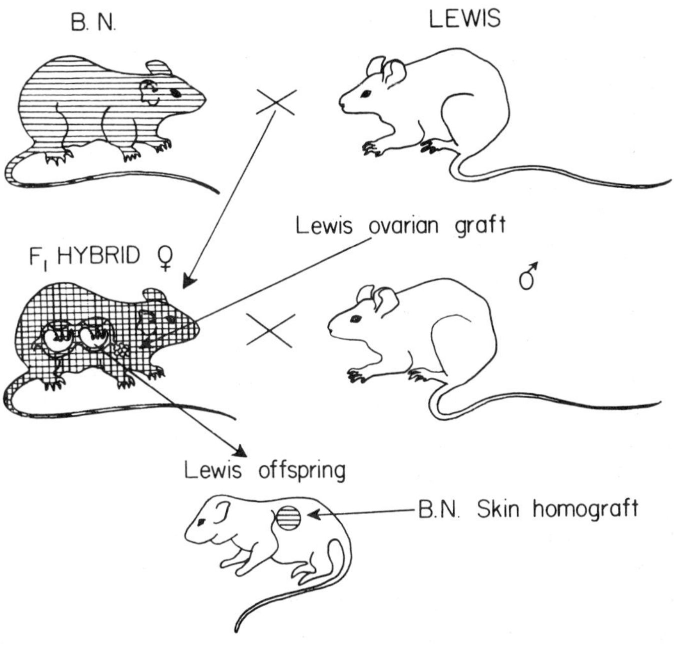

Fig. 12.4. Experimental design for determining whether there is a natural exposure of rats to maternal transplantation antigens.

mothers, had an opportunity to become "infiltrated" by F_1 (BN antigen-bearing) cells. When these animals were three days old, they were grafted with BN skin. None of them gave evidence of being tolerant, but some of them rejected their grafts faster than control hosts did, which suggested that they had been sensitized, possibly as a consequence of exposure to very small dosages of F_1 cells (see Chapter 10). This may have occurred at the time of parturition.

In man, an interesting claim of possible clinical significance was made, by Dr. Lyndon Peer and his associates, that children will frequently accept skin grafts from their mothers for much longer periods than they will accept grafts from their fathers. This work still awaits independent confirmation. However, there is a strong prima facie case that maternally induced tolerance does occur naturally in the case of one highly invasive tumor, malignant melanoma. There are at least five cases on record in which women suffering from this disease during pregnancy have given birth to offspring who subsequently developed and succumbed to this tumor within a few months of birth. It is surprising, in the light of this evidence, that leukemia is not transmitted in this manner since, in this disease, malignant cells are certainly present in the maternal blood stream.

Attempts to Increase the Permeability of the Placental Barrier to Cells

Several attempts have been made to increase the permeability of the placental barrier to cells by experimental artifice and so obtain a more impressive degree of maternally induced tolerance. In appropriately designed experiments Lengerová, and Ramseier and Brent, independently, have shown that *local* irradiation of the uterine horns or placentas of pregnant rats may lead to the induction of tolerance of their mother's skin grafts in a significant proportion of the offspring. In rabbits there have been two reports that the administration of hyaluronidase and/or histamine to pregnant females partially or even completely abrogates the ability of a significant proportion of their offspring to reject grafts of maternal skin. Of greater interest is the report that some females subjected to this treatment subsequently proved to be tolerant of their offsprings' skin grafts.

Recently Drs. Tuffrey, Bishun, and Barnes of London have reported findings which suggested a very high maternal $\longrightarrow$ fetal traffic in cells in the mouse. They took female CBA mice, homozygous for the T_6 chromosome marker, and mated them with CBA (T_6T_6) males. Two and a half days later, fertilized eggs from inbred CFW mice, which do not have the T_6 marker, were transferred to the uterine horns of the previously mated CBA females. The resulting mixed litters (the CFW members could be distinguished by their color) were killed four to sixty days postpartum, and various tissues including bone marrow and lymphoid tissues were examined cytologically. It was reported that 3 to 30% of alien (T_6T_6)-labeled cells were present among the dividing cells examined. Although the authors conceded that these cells might have been acquired from their CBA siblings in utero, they felt that the cells were of maternal origin. In a subsequent study in which, with the aid of the same chromosome marker, evidence of cell chimerism due to immigration of maternal cells was sought in hybrid offspring, chimerism proved to be very infrequent. However, a careful attempt on the part of four independent groups of investigators has failed to confirm these findings. It does not, however, exclude the possibility that the CFW mice used by Tuffrey and her colleagues were unusual in the extent to which they allowed the passage of cells from mother to fetus.

Does Homologous or Transplantation Disease Ever Occur Naturally?

As mentioned in Chapter 11, if a sufficient number of immunologically competent cells from adult donors are injected into very young (fetal or perinatal) homologous avian or mammalian hosts, runt disease or transplantation disease may result. Soon after it had been shown that peripheral blood contains immunologically competent cells among its small lymphocyte moiety, attention was drawn to the possibility that runt disease might sometimes occur naturally if enough maternal leucocytes gained access to a genetically appropriate fetus.

Since 1965 a few cases of XX/XY mosaicism in the blood of infants or abortuses have been reported which appear to be due to prenatal entry of maternal (XX) cells into the circulation of male fetuses. In one of these, symptoms highly suggestive of runt disease were described.

In considering the possible outcome of naturally transmitted low dosages of maternal cells on the fetus, it is important to recognize that in some species, including man and sheep, there is evidence of the acquisition of immunological competence to some antigens long before birth. For example, fetal sheep can react against skin homografts transplanted to them at mid-gestation, i.e., at about seventy-five days before birth, and human fetuses can respond to some microbial antigens during the third and possibly during the latter part of the second trimester. Thus the ability to destroy relatively small numbers of immigrant maternal cells may also be developed at an early stage and may account for the rarity of transmission of malignant disease.

In both rats and mice, it was once generally believed that, if inoculation of neonatal subjects with homologous cells did anything at all, it induced tolerance. However, several studies have shown that the introduction of relatively small numbers of cells at this time of life may result in a weak, transient state of sensitivity. How soon before birth they are capable of becoming sensitized remains to be determined.

Also relevant to this discussion are findings of Dr. J. Dancis and his associates which suggest that immunologically competent cells are present in mouse placenta which are capable of GVH reactivity and antibody synthesis. However, the cell type responsible has not yet been identified. The possibility that fetal leucocytes present in the placental tissue are the active agents remains on probation. It is perhaps pertinent that Dr. A. M. Silverstein finds evidence of immunological competence in fetal sheep before overt evidence of lymphoid tissue differentiation. The possession of immunologic function *within* the placenta might well confer survival advantage upon mammals, protecting them against the hazards of microbial infection from their mothers and also from the risk of developing runt disease.

Teleologically, Nature had to find a solution to the homograft problem as an essential prerequisite for embarking upon the evolution of the mammals, i.e., to minimize the immunologic hazard of being gestated. Her solution has proved to be almost perfect. It is unfortunate that it does not lend itself to clinical application in overcoming host resistance to organ homografts.

REFERENCES

Billingham, R. E. 1964. Transplantation immunity and the maternal-fetal relation. New Eng. J. Med. 270:667–672; 720–725.

Lanman, J. T. 1965. Transplantation immunity in mammalian pregnancy; mechanisms of fetal protection against immunologic rejection. J. Pediat. 66:525–540.

Kirby, D. R. S. 1968. Transplantation and pregnancy, pp. 565–586. *In* F. T. Rapaport and J. Dausset [ed.] Human transplantation. Grune and Stratton, New York.

Chapter 13

Immunosuppression

Interest in the suppression of immunological responses has increased rapidly over the past two decades, motivated by the desire to discover or develop means of abrogating host reactivity to therapeutic homografts, to treat immunologic diseases, and to study the kinetics of immune responses at the cellular level.

As long ago as 1916, the immunosuppressive properties of benzene and toluene were under investigation. Benzene was found to impair the capacity of rabbits to produce antibodies against sheep erythrocytes, and Dr. Ludvig Hektoen of Chicago correctly concluded that this substance affects the cellular elements responsible for antibody synthesis. The observation made during World War I that mustard gas killed its victims by destroying bone marrow and lymphoid tissue soon led to the discovery of the immunosuppressive properties of dichloroethylsufide in dogs, rats, and other animals.

The capacity of X-irradiation, even when given repeatedly in small dosages, to weaken an animal's resistance to tumor homografts by almost selectively destroying its lymphoid tissues was well established in the 1920s. It has long been known that certain colloidal substances, such as the dye trypan blue and thorotrast, can weaken a host's response to tumor homografts, as can intraperitoneal injections of olive oil.

As Medawar has recently pointed out, immunosuppressive agents are so varied in their characters and in their modes of action, so far as these are known, that no rational classification is possible. Two important agents which, under appropriate conditions, may exert powerful immunosuppressant effects have already been discussed in detail:

1. *Antibody* which, if administered *prior* to exposure to an appropriate type of homograft, may inhibit the host's response in the phenomenon known as immunological enhancement (see Chapter 7).
2. *Antigen* which, if appropriately administered, may induce a specific

state of immunological unresponsiveness known as tolerance or paralysis (see Chapter 10).

In addition to these immunosuppressive agents, the following include the "conventional" immunosuppressants:

3. *Cytotoxic and Antiproliferative Agents.* This broad category includes ionizing irradiation; alkylating agents such as nitrogen and sulfur mustards; phosphoramides such as cyclophosphamide and chlorambucil; antagonists of folic acid such as aminopterin, amethopterin, and methotrexate; purine and pyrimidine analogues (sometimes called fraudulent bases) including 6-mercaptopurine and a derivative, azothioprine (known as Imuran, the standard immunosuppressive drug used in clinical transplantation); methylhydrazine derivatives; antibiotics such as actinomycin, mitomycin, and chloramphenicol; and certain plant alkaloids.

The first demonstration of the capacity of whole-body X-irradiation to prolong the lives of homografts of *normal* tissue was made in 1950 by Drs. Dempster, Lennox, and Boag in London. They showed that the survival time of skin homografts in rabbits was almost doubled by prior exposure of the hosts to a sublethal dosage of 250 r. In 1955 came the demonstration that irradiation facilitated the establishment of bone marrow grafts of alien origin. In 1958 attempts began at several centers to use whole-body irradiation as the immunosuppressant for human renal transplantation. Although a few long-term survivals resulted with kidney grafts from living related donors, there were so many failures that it soon became evident that a better means of immunosuppression was required. However, it is still standard practice to apply irradiation *locally* to renal homografts when rejection crises threaten their well-being.

In 1959 Drs. Robert Schwartz and William Dameshek, in Boston, made the important discovery that, when rabbits were injected with human serum albumin followed by daily injections of 6-mercaptopurine (6-MP), their immunological response to this immunogen was blocked, the animals becoming tolerant. A year later these workers demonstrated that this drug could triple the survival time of skin homografts on rabbits. In 1960 Dr. Roy Calne in England and, subsequently, other investigators demonstrated the capacity of 6-MP to prolong the survival of renal homografts in dogs. Within the next two years, collaborative work by Dr. Calne and Dr. Joseph Murray at the Peter Brent Brigham Hospital, Boston, and Dr. George Hitchings of the Wellcome Laboratories resulted in the development of a related but less toxic drug, azathioprine (Imuran), which had the added advantage that it could be administered orally instead of by injection. In 1963 this drug was successfully employed clinically, and it still remains the most widely used drug for clinical immunosuppression.

Most of the agents listed at the beginning of this section (see also Table 13.1) were introduced into medical practice primarily as chemo-

Table 13.1

Some immunosuppressant drugs and their modes of action

Type of drug	*Examples*	*Mode of action*
Alkylating agents (= radiomimetic drugs)	Nitrogen and Sulfur Mustards Cyclophosphamide (Cytoxan) Chlorambucil, Myleran Methylhydrazine	Highly reactive with nucleophilic centers in molecules. Probably inhibit many enzyme systems as well as affecting DNA by combining with it. Highly cytotoxic, have profound affects on lymphoid and myeloid tissues. May arrest cells in premitotic (G-2) phase of cell cycle.
Folic acid antagonists	Aminopterin, Amethopterin (Methotrexate)	Interfere with conversion of folic acid to tetrafolinic acid needed for synthesis of purine and thymine. Thus block synthesis of DNA and RNA and purine-containing enzymes. Potent inhibitors of mitosis.
Purine and pyrimidine analogues	6-Mercaptopurine (6-MP) Thioguanine Azathioprine (Imuran)	Affect synthesis and interconversion of purine nucleotides so that they may inhibit synthesis of nucleic acids and of purine-containing enzymes.
Antibiotics	Actinomycin C and D Chloramphenicol	Inhibit RNA synthesis by combining with DNA.
	Mitomycin	Depolmyerizes and cross-links DNA, inhibiting its replication.

therapeutic agents against cancer. In no sense can their immunosuppressive properties be regarded as specific. Their capacity to inhibit immunological responses is simply a consequence of their generalized toxic influence upon dividing cells of *all* kinds, and the fact that mitotic activity on the part of antigen-stimulated cells is an essential component of all immunological responses. Evidence for this important conclusion was presented by Brent and Medawar. They found that none of these agents had any discernible influence on the initial stages of either the NLT reaction or the ILT reaction in guinea pigs' skin (see Chapter 8), whether administered to the cell donors *before* the lymphocytes were harvested for transfer, to the cells in vitro while in transit from donor to recipient, or to the host. These workers argue very cogently that the immunosuppressive activity of these agents depends upon their interference with the amplification of the immune response, which takes place through proliferation of antigen-stimulated cells *after* the initial recognition event has occurred.

It must be emphasized that most, if not all, of the agents in the present category inhibit immunities mediated by antibodies to a greater extent than they inhibit immunities mediated by cells. It is this fact that makes immunosuppression so difficult for the clinician to manage, especially in the case of patients with badly mismatched organ homografts. They need enough of the agent to inhibit graft rejection, yet not so much as to deprive them of their natural defenses against pathogenic infections. In practice, although immunosuppressive therapy is never discontinued, in most successful cases the maintenance dosage is ultimately reduced to a reasonably harmless level. This is probably due in part to the induction of some degree of immunological tolerance in the host in conjunction with the processes that underlie the phenomenon of adaptation on the part of the graft (see Chapter 6).

4. *Steroids.* Despite the optimism raised by the initial discovery in 1951 that the adrenal corticosteroid hormone, cortisone, weakens the reactivity of rabbits against skin homografts, the immunosuppressant capacity of this agent and related natural or synthetic compounds soon proved to be too weak for their employment as primary immunosuppressants. However, unlike the other agents considered so far, chronically administered steroids at relatively high dosage levels are capable of abrogating an extant state of transplantation sensitivity. Because of this property they are employed clinically to help reverse rejection crises. Exactly how steroids prevent sensitized lymphocytes from destroying homografts is still a matter of conjecture. Most authorities believe that they inhibit the nonspecific inflammatory component of the homograft reaction. In addition it has been suggested that they may delay the recruitment and/or deployment of lymphocytes into the recirculating pool (see Chapter 8).

5. *Ribonuclease.* In 1959 Dr. Benjamin Kamrin discovered that an alpha globulin fraction of serum was capable of prolonging the survival of skin homografts in rats. Subsequently, in 1963, Dr. J. F. Mowbray reported that fraction C of normal bovine serum has immunosuppressive properties, almost certainly due to a ribonuclease in the alpha 2-glycoprotein fraction. Later work revealed that pancreatic ribonuclease had similar immunosuppressive properties, provided that it was first linked to an appropriate carrier protein. This agent has been shown to impair the response of dogs to renal homografts, and of mice to H-2 incompatible skin grafts. When administered to adult mice, in conjunction with homologous lymphoid cells, it abets the induction of some degree of tolerance. It seems to be relatively harmless and is believed to act by interfering with the early stages of the immune response.

6. *Colloidal Dyes.* The previously mentioned capacity of colloidal dyes, such as trypan blue, to weaken homograft reactivity still awaits systematic investigation. The conventional explanation of their mode of action is that they "blockade" the reticuloendothelial system.

7. *Antilymphocyte Serum (ALS).* This has been under episodic investigation since it was first employed in 1899 by the famous Russian zoologist, Elie Metchnikoff, in his studies on macrophages. Its capacity to

interfere with the homograft reaction was first demonstrated by Woodruff and Anderson in 1963.

ALS is raised in animals of one species by injecting them with lymphoid cells from donors of the species in which it is to be employed. For example, ALS for use in mice is normally prepared by injecting murine lymphoid cells into rabbits, and ALS for human use is usually raised in horses. The genetic constitution of the donor of the cells employed is completely immaterial.

The results obtained with ALS in laboratory rodents are truly dramatic in terms of the degree of prolongation of the lives of tissue and organ homografts and even *heterografts* obtainable.

The various immunosuppressive agents just described all have serious shortcomings largely because, in addition to unwanted side effects, they are not specifically immunosuppressive and impair humoral immunities to a greater degree than they impair cellular immunities. However, ALS (especially its immunologically effective component, the IgG fraction of the antiserum) has proved to be relatively harmless and nontoxic at the dosage levels required to hold homograft reactivity in abeyance. It also acts *more* effectively against cellular immunities than against humoral immunities. For example, Drs. Lance and Batchelor have shown that H-2 locus incompatible skin homografts, surviving on mice under the protection of ALS, eventually elicit the formation of relatively high titers of specific antibodies in spite of complete abrogation of the homograft reaction.

Unlike nearly all other immunosuppressants, ALS has the capacity to abolish a preexisting state of sensitivity against homografts, i.e., of erasing immunological memory when administered at high dosage levels. Furthermore, its effectiveness in abrogating a host's reactivity to alien grafts is much less dependent upon the magnitude of the immunogenetic disparity involved, than is the case with other immunosuppressants.

Two important properties which ALS shares with other immunosuppressive agents are: first, it will facilitate the induction of tolerance in adult hosts concomitantly inoculated with donor lymphoid cells; second, its effect is usually augmented and prolonged by thymectomy.

Although numerous hypotheses concerning the mode of action of ALS have been advanced and explored experimentally, it is now more-or-less generally agreed that it acts principally if not entirely by the complement-dependent, selective killing of the thymus-derived population of long-lived lymphocytes of the recirculating pool. Since it contains a complex of foreign proteins, ALS is strongly antigenic. However, this property, which clinically can have deleterious effects, may be avoided by previously rendering the host tolerant of normal gamma globulin from the ALS-donating species.

So far, ALS raised in horses has been used only as an adjunct to the conventional immunosuppressant procedures in man. However, even with the relatively low dosages employed (as compared with the much higher dosages used in experimental animals), striking improvements in the results of renal and hepatic transplants have been reported. Many different laboratories and pharmaceutical companies are now engaged in the large-scale production of ALS for therapeutic application, and strenuous efforts are being made to devise a simple means of assaying its activity.

ALS and Heterografts

Throughout the history of transplantation there have been many small-scale attempts to employ heterografts (or xenografts) for clinical or experimental purposes, almost all of which have been totally unsuccessful. Unlike homografts, grafts exchanged between members of *different* species rarely become established to the point where they begin to fulfill their normal function. Indeed, they may scarcely be said to have any meaningful survival time at all. The few exceptions include grafts exchanged between species that are closely related taxonomically, such as birds of the Order Galliformes (chickens, turkeys, pheasants, guinea fowl, etc.); golden hamsters (*Mesocricetus auratus auratus*) and a wild hamster species (*Mesocricetus auratus brandti*); and sheep and goats. The fate of heterografts exchanged between members of such species as these closely resembles that of homografts.

Worthy of comment at this stage are the results of attempts to use renal heterografts in heavily immunosuppressed patients. Although baboon kidneys in man thrived longer than one might have anticipated, the results were disappointing clinically. With chimpanzees as donors, however, Dr. Keith Reemtsma and his associates have had patients living for as long as nine months.

Hitherto the results of most attempts in the laboratory to overcome the incompatibility of heterografts, by inoculation of very young hosts with donor cells or by attempts to rehabilitate lethally irradiated hosts with heterologous bone marrow cell infusions, have given very disappointing results. Nevertheless, rat ⟶ mouse radiation chimeras have been produced.

Now, thanks to ALS, heterografts are beginning to capture the imagination and attention of transplanters. Chronic ALS treatment will enable grafts of rat skin to survive on mice or hamsters for many months; grafts of skin from guinea pigs, rabbits, and even man to live on mice for a long time; or grafts of sheep or goat skin to live on calves for many weeks.

More exciting is the prospect of tolerance-induction across the hitherto seemingly inviolable species barriers. Lance and his associates have recently shown that adult mice can be rendered tolerant of grafts of rat skin by what is admittedly a rather heroic procedure. This entails thymectomy, followed by a short but intensive period of treatment with ALS, and a massive infusion of rat lymphoid cells (100×10^6). To eliminate the intervention of graft-versus-host reactions (see Chapter 11), the lymphoid cell donors were treated with ALS beforehand. Tolerant mice produced in this way were found to be chimeric with respect to their lymphoid cells and manufactured rat proteins.

The fact that ALS prolongs the survival of heterografts and facilitates the induction of tolerance with respect to them affords formal proof that, at least with the particular donor/host species combinations concerned, the failure of heterografts to thrive on untreated subjects is the outcome of an immunological process, rather than something more fundamental, such as inability of the host to supply an essential metabolite.

Clearly, we can't make generalizations about heterografts. Even with a particular donor/host species combination, there may be special problems relating to particular tissues and organs, especially those that synthesize distinctive secretory products which may themselves incite specific immunological responses. With different species, the conditions required to overcome heterograft incompatibility may vary considerably—there are probably "good" and "bad" combinations. Furthermore, with some combinations, heterograft rejection may well be principally a cell-mediated phenomenon, whereas with others, antibodies may be the prime movers of the rejection process. There are also grounds for suspecting that eosinophils may play a role in the resistance to heterografts.

ALS indicates the feasibility of developing synthetic agents which, without any generalized toxic reactions, will suppress cellular immunities perhaps even more effectively. However, some of our defenses against microbial pathogens are cell-mediated, and there is an increasing body of evidence which points to the existence of a cell-mediated tumor surveillance mechanism, whose normal functioning will obviously be impaired by chronic treatments with agents like ALS that impair cellular immunities nonspecifically. Therefore, some means of obviating chronic therapy of any kind is needed. The ultimate solution to the homograft (and heterograft) problem almost certainly lies in a simple and reproducible means of inducing a *specific* impairment of the pertinent segment of the host's repertoire of immunologic responses, i.e., the induction of tolerance.

It is interesting to note that surgeons are already becoming aware of an abnormally high incidence of malignant lymphomas in recipients of renal homografts who have been chronically immunosuppressed. Of course, there is as yet no proof that this is the outcome of interference with a normal tumor surveillance mechanism(s).

The prospects of being able to solve the logistic problems of organ transplantation by resort to heterografts are now very bright, and the old metaphoric concept of the sheep in wolf's clothing could probably be translated into reality if such an animal would fulfill any useful purpose.

REFERENCES

Lance, E. M., R. H. Levey, P. B. Medawar, and M. Ruszkiewicz. 1969. Tolerance of rat skin grafts in adult mice. Nat. Acad. Sci. (Washington), Proc. 64:1356–1361.

Ludford, R. J. 1931. Resistance to the growth of transplantable tumors. II. The influence of dyestuffs and of colloids on natural resistance. Brit. J. Exp. Pathol. 12:108–113.

Medawar, P. B. 1968. Biological effects of heterologous antilymphocyte sera, p. 501–509. *In* F. T. Rapaport and J. Dausset [ed.]. Human transplantation. Grune and Stratton, New York.

Medawar, P. B. 1969. Antilymphocytic serum: its properties and potential. Hosp. Prac. 5:26–33.

Medawar, P. B. 1969. Immunosuppressive agents, with special reference to antilymphocyte serum. Roy. Soc. (London), Proc., B. 174:155–172.

Reemtsma, K. 1968. Heterotransplantation, p. 357–366. *In* F. T. Rapaport and J. Dausset [ed.]. Human transplantation. Grune and Stratton, New York.

Schwartz, R. S. 1968. Immunosuppressive drug therapy, p. 440–471. *In* F. T. Rapaport and J. Dausset [ed.]. Human transplantation. Grune and Stratton, New York.

Smith, L. H. and C. C. Congdon. 1968. Biological effects of ionizing radiation, p. 510–525. *In* F. T. Rapaport and J. Dausset [ed.]. Human transplantation. Grune and Stratton, New York.

General References

GENERAL REFERENCES

Van Bekkum, D. W., and M. J. de Vries. 1967. Radiation chimeras. Academic Press, New York.

Billingham, R. E., and W. K. Silvers [ed.]. 1961. Transplantation of tissues and cells. Wistar Press, Philadelphia, Pa.

Burnet, F. M. 1969. Cellular immunology. Cambridge University Press, London.

Elves, M. W. 1966. The lymphocytes. Lippincott Co., Philadelphia, Pa.

Hildemann, W. H. 1970. Immunogenetics. Holden-Day, San Francisco.

Holborow, E. J. 1968. An ABC of Modern Immunology. Little, Brown and Co., Boston, Mass.

Landy, M., and W. Braun [ed.]. 1969. Immunological tolerance. Academic Press, New York.

Lawrence, H. S., and M. Landy [ed.]. 1969. Mediators of cellular immunity. Academic Press, New York.

Lengerová, A. 1969. Immunogenetics of tissue transplantation. John Wiley & Sons, Inc., New York.

Micklem, H. S., and J. F. Loutit. 1966. Tissue grafting and radiation. Academic Press, New York.

Möller, G. [ed.]. 1969. Antigen-sensitive cells. Transpl. Rev. 1. The Williams and Wilkins Co., Baltimore, Maryland.

Rapaport, F. T., and J. Dausset [ed.]. 1968. Human transplantation. Grune and Stratton, New York.

Russell, P. S., and A. P. Monaco. 1965. The biology of tissue transplantation. Little, Brown and Co., Boston, Mass.

Russell, P. S. and H. J. Winn. 1970. Transplantation. New Eng. J. Med. 282:786–793, 848–854, 896–906.

Samter, M. [ed.]. 1965. Immunological diseases. Little, Brown and Co., Boston, Mass.

Woodruff, M. F. A. 1960. The transplantation of tissues and organs. Charles C. Thomas, Springfield, Illinois.

Index

C

D

E

F

G

H

I

J

K

L

M

N

O

P

R

T

U

W

X

Y

Z